Diabetes
DANGER

Diabetes
DANGER

What 200 Million Americans at Risk Need to Know

Walter M. Bortz II, M.D.

SelectBooks, Inc.

First Edition
ISBN 1-59079-103-7

Library of Congress Cataloging-in-Publication Data

Bortz, Walter M.
Diabetes danger : what 200 million Americans at risk need to know /
Walter M. Bortz II.-- 1st ed.
     p. cm.
Includes index.
ISBN 1-59079-103-7 (hardcover : alk. paper)
1. Diabetes. 2. Consumer education. I. Title.

RC660.B65 2005
616.4'62--dc22

2005024122

Manufactured in the United States of America

10 9 8 7 6 5 4 3 2 1

Anyone who pokes around the details of a disaster inevitably finds heroes and heroines, people who labor mightily to reduce the damage done.

When considering who might qualify for the valor medal winners in the current diabetes disaster, I immediately identify the thousands of health workers, those who struggle daily to extinguish the diabetes inferno. These workers have varied types of training, experiences and duties. However, they all share in an earnest effort of lightening the burden of the millions of persons with diabetes or those prone to the disease. Among these are the diabetes educators, whose role is absolutely critical: nutritionists, nurses, exercise trainers, psychologists, and physician extenders of different types.

Your work, which sometimes may seem like rolling large stones up a hill, lacks glamour, but is truly valiant.

I offer you my thanks. And with deep appreciation, I dedicate this book to you.

Contents

Acknowledgments

In the joint effort which this book represents I acknowledge with thanks, first, Kathy Gold, RN, MSN, CDE, my colleague at Diabetes Research and Wellness Foundation (DRWF), whose clinical skills and knowledge are closely matched by her editorial guidance. I would also like to thank Mike Gretschel, volunteer president; Andi Gretschel-Stancik, executive director; John Alahouzos, Chairman of the Diabetes Research and Wellness Foundation Board of Directors. The Board of Directors have also been steadfast in their support and delivery of this book. I would like to recognize these individuals for their overwhelming support of diabetes research and their efforts through the foundation to keep individuals with diabetes healthy until a cure is found.

Dana Isaacson of SelectBooks has been a skillful and even inspired editor.

I thank Jeffrey and Donna Wyant, whose extensive efforts made this book a reality.

I acknowledge Rhett Currier for her tender and terrible family tale. She tells the story of the book more powerfully than I ever could have.

I thank Governor Mike Huckabee for his involvement with the book. Political leadership that he provides offers bright hope among the grim headlines which dominate most news about diabetes.

I acknowledge the Health Trust for providing space and time for this effort. Of course, I thank my family for their interest and indulgence.

Finally, I thank my patients for allowing me to share in their lives, and learn with and from them the evils of diabetes.

Prologue

By Rhett Currier

My parents were like Romeo and Juliet, Napoleon and Josephine, or Ricky and Lucy. Dad made a great life with Mom as his partner—despite his diabetes. He had three tow-headed kids, a smart, gorgeous wife, and was a full professor with an endowed chair at the University of Virginia Law School at the age of 35. He then left teaching and built a lucrative practice on Wall Street, making the formerly boring practice of municipal bonds sexy by inventing something called "advanced refunding." Mom and Dad kept his diabetes a secret from clients; if they knew, Dad feared clients would not hire him.

Later, when the United States Supreme Court cited my brilliant father's scholarly work, Dad could not read it because of the devastating stroke caused by diabetes. The stroke had not been strong enough to kill, but he had never recovered from it. He lived the rest of his life in diapers, unable to walk, feed or bathe himself. His speech was slurred, one side paralyzed, his hand frozen in place. He recognized close friends and family, people who meant something to him. Most of the time, though, his mind was in shadows—he would ask for his father who had died 25 years before. I would tell him Grandfather was at the office. If I didn't lie, Dad cried upon learning of his father's death. Dad would say over and over to "Go! Go! Go!" (presumably for a roll in his wheelchair). He would shout out over and over "Help! Help!" And he would say my mother's name over and over again: "Barbara, help!"

Dad's brain would rewire itself and he would then have rare lucid moments, wonderful respites when he was able to escape the prison of his injured brain. From his wheelchair in a child's playground where I had taken him outside of the hospital, he looked into my eyes. His eyes were clear: my Dad was there. He said "I'm sorry I got this way, I didn't mean for it to happen. Please tell Mom I'm so sorry." I told him he had nothing to apologize for, it was not his fault. It was diabetes' fault.

When one person in the family has diabetes, you all have it. I bet my Mom saved my father's life 1,500 times in 37 years. About once a week, something happened. One morning, Mom was going to let Dad sleep in (as she was off to an early Bible group study). She tweaked his toe to say bye to his horizontal body, and through the sheet she felt cold sweat. He was passed out, in shock. Her hands shaking—you never get used to the emergencies—she filled a syringe to inject him with glucagon, and brought him back from the edge. If she hadn't tweaked his toe, he would have died.

Dad was diagnosed with diabetes two days after my eldest brother Ford was born. Ford was diagnosed with diabetes at age 2½. Mom knew what it meant. She had been a biochemistry double major, and had forgone medical school to marry Dad and raise a family. When Ford was born, the doctors told my parents to have more children because this one wouldn't make it through high school.

Both Mom and Dad learned to give injections. Dad gave them to himself, and later Ford was taught to inject himself. You have to get it right; if you screw up, your kid dies. How do you explain the syringe to your kid, how do you promise him a normal life? Ford could spend the night at my grandparents, because my grandmother Caroline was not afraid to learn to give injections. He could also spend the night at another diabetic kid's house.

When I was seven, I woke up hearing thumping, screaming and shouting. I catapulted out of bed and into the hallway. Mom hovered over Ford. He was writhing, hitting the walls with his hands and feet and making a screaming, gurgling sound.

Mom shouted to my brother. "Tom, get the glucagon on my night table! Fill up the syringe!" Tom was ten then, had never filled the syringe before, but he had watched often enough to do it right.

"Rhett!" she cried to me. "Go get Dr. Tirk! Now!"

I ran from the house, hopped onto my Stingray bicycle and rode as fast as I could go to fetch the doctor. I had never been more scared.

Mom gave Ford the injection, and he went to the hospital. When he came home he was sick to his stomach, staying on the couch for a day or two. Ford was angry, saying Mom had given him too much glucagon. Hey, better than croaking. That summer, Ford had a diabetic reaction about once a week.

When Ford lived with a friend after college, the friend called up my parents because Ford was acting weird, eating cigarette butts. Ford was in shock, on autopilot: he could not see, could not hear, he was just grabbing at something to eat to bring his blood sugar up. Mom told the friend to give Ford a sugary soda, and his blood sugar was raised.

Ford had a crush on a cute girl, so I invited her to a dinner party we were having. Ford did not want the girl to know about the diabetes; I saw him adjust his insulin pump under the table where she could not see it. Sometime later, I noticed Ford's dilated pupils, and I thought he was going into shock. I asked quietly if he was okay, and he claimed too firmly that he was fine. This, of course, meant he was in shock. Since Ford was in denial mode because of the cute girl, I lured the whole crowd into the kitchen and parked Ford in front of our always-abundant supply of chocolate candies. On autopilot, he chewed. Blood sugar returning to normal, Ford was happy the cute girl never caught on.

For no real reason, my brother Tom stopped at my parents' house one midday—Ford had moved back home after college. Tom found Ford passed out on the floor, facedown in a diabetic coma. Tom saved his life.

Watching Dad die, Ford witnessed how diabetes would later kill him. Ford wanted to do everything to keep Dad alive, hoping Dad would recover enough faculties to be able to enjoy his life. But month after month, we watched the cycle: Dad's brain re-circuiting, his realization of how screwed up he was, the emotional panic which would trigger another stroke.

A series of strokes took away Dad's ability to speak. We brought him home after 6 months in the hospital. But stroke victims don't sleep and Mom could hear Dad crying out to her in the night, Barbara, Help! ... but she couldn't. More strokes came, and Dad took no notice of anyone around him for several weeks. He became a vegetable who looked like my handsome Dad. We had talked about letting Dad die by withholding his insulin, but none of us wanted to do that—even though it seemed more humane than letting him live like that, especially when Dad's living will provided otherwise. I prayed that my Dad would no longer be tortured by this life he was barely living. And that prayer was answered: Dad died and we were all there with him.

I know that he is in an infinitely better place after living a slow-motion death. I could not have imagined a worse death ... until I watched my brother's death. Ford died over a ten-year plus period. He had kidney failure at 25, and the dialysis caused an infection that led to a huge weight loss. My brother stood at 5 feet 11 inches, at 120 pounds with an open pit in his stomach where they let the wound drain, as they worked to get rid of an infection. We took turns in Ford's hospital room so he would never be alone. I would go in the afternoon after my college courses were done to relieve Mom, Caroline or Tom—we took our shifts.

Later that summer, on the day that Prince Charles and Diana got married, my brother Tom donated one of his kidneys to Ford at the University of Minnesota Hospital. They told Ford his life expectancy was five years. But using one of the world's first insulin pumps, the transplanted kidney lasted longer than Charles and Diana's marriage. Tom still feels the pain whenever he coughs—at the site where they cut open his torso so he could give his kidney to Ford.

Ford made good use of Tom's kidney. He graduated from Columbia University, got married and became a teacher. He took a counseling degree from New York University and became an AIDS hospice counselor, just as AIDS was being accepted as a medical epidemic. Who better than a diabetic like Ford to understand what it is like to face your own mortality?

But diabetes clogged Ford's heart, and it went misdiagnosed as depression. His marriage fell apart. Having been declared disabled by Social Security, he moved in with my Grandmother Caroline. After Caroline's death, Ford's new lady-friend (Ford was a charmer like his Dad, and always had a lady-friend looking after him) figured out Ford was having silent heart attacks. Then Mom convinced them to go to Minnesota where the transplant had been done. At age 39, Ford had a quintuple bypass, and the next year he had a kidney pancreas transplant.

He was 40 years old and was dependent, sick, uninsured and unable to work. He was also smart, determined, and expected to beat the odds—and he was lucky enough to have some independent means, a supportive lady-friend and a caring family and friends.

No longer diabetic, some damage could repair itself. The numbness in his hands and feet faded, and he stopped getting hemorrhages in his eyes that clouded his vision. The nerve and heart damage was irreversible. His hands would shake, and his heart was weakened.

Ford re-engaged in society, writing a much-talked-about, increasingly provocative opinion column for the local newspaper. His romantic relationship fell apart as the manic depressive episodes caused by the anti-rejection medications made him difficult to handle. He would be up, then normal, then down. The cycles became more pronounced as did the behavior. His social relationships were greatly challenged. Some folks didn't get that he was ill; they just thought he was quirky. But with his gregarious nature and unrelenting determination to beat diabetes, Ford sought out a circle of understanding friends. They were all a bit quirky too!

With the mania, the medications also induced a cyclical paranoia, which grew increasingly pronounced. Fear made Ford reclusive. He lived with a fear that was all too real to him, and I could not reason him out of it. I thought about having him declared insane, but I did not want to see him institutionalized nor could I take care of him myself. And what would that do but humiliate him, and take away the independence that meant so much? And Ford had a great ability to flip the switch and act like everything was fine.

Finally, Paul, Ford's best pal from college, visited. Paul witnessed the paranoia, but he also saw that Ford was still there: Ford would switch off the paranoia talk, and then they'd get into an intellectual discussion about politics, the Yankees or the Shreveport Mudbugs hockey team. Paul helped Ford realize he was suffering from paranoia, and Ford sought treatment.

But the paranoia medication destroyed Ford's pancreas function, and he again became diabetic. In the Shreveport hospital, Ford's condition worsened. His doctor agreed with Mom; it was time to take Ford to Minnesota. Since Ford could not sit up, I hired an air ambulance—basically a flying ICU with a nurse (you can look it up in the yellow pages). Ford was ready to give up, fearing his kidney and pancreas were shutting down for good. He was defeated, ready to die.

But a former flame told Ford he was going to Minnesota, and when I explained how easy the air ambulance would be—with room for the nurse, me, Mom and the former flame—Ford believed he could beat the odds again. And he did. Ford's kidney function returned, but his pancreas failed. He became diabetic once again—a complete nightmare. My Mom moved in with him, and for six months nursed him back to health, awaiting another pancreas transplant.

His fourth transplant was tough. Mom stayed in a nearby hotel; Tom, cousins Denise and Jimmy and I each would visit to lend support to Ford and to Mom. Ford battled an infection for two months, and was finally released. Mom, with the help of Minnesota friends Ryan and Julie, took Ford to our childhood summer house in Nantucket. Ford had a glorious time. I think he knew it was likely his last time there.

At the invitation of Ryan and Julie, Ford returned to live what was to be his last year in Minnesota, near the hospital. Ford's home with Ryan, Julie and later, Ben was like a dorm, lots of interaction—it was more fun to be with the tribe than hang out with your Mommy. They gave Ford a feeling of normalcy. Mom would still visit to check on everyone.

Several weeks after the move, Ford had his first rejection episode, and he struggled to recover. Then his kidney failed and he again had to report for dialysis three times a week. His heart needed another kidney transplant, and they had to wait a few weeks until he was stable enough to handle it. The medications made him sleep all the time, especially the new heart medications. The weather grew colder and the winter nights longer and darker. Ford needed a new kidney, and he knew I would give him mine if his body qualified as a viable transplant candidate. But his heart was in terrible shape; diabetes destroys your circulatory system. And it destroys your electrical system. Ford was subject to sudden collapse—his legs would just give away.

Getting ready to go for dialysis, Ford turned blue. Blood gushed from his nose. He was rushed to the hospital and was on life support until the family gathered—his Minnesota family and his birth family.

We circled his ICU bed, each with a hand on a part of him. His broad shoulders and hands were puffy from hospital stays, his foot missing toes from an amputation. When they stopped injecting him with medication to keep his heart pumping, Ford lived another hour and a half. His heart kept fighting back just as he'd done all of his life. We could not believe that Ford had not been able to beat the odds this time, that now, he was dying.

Ford had not reached his 49th birthday.

Foreword

Governor Mike Huckabee of Arkansas

There was always a gaggle of reporters waiting for me at the top of the steps, I knew they'd have a question for me and I'd pray it was a long one, because I knew I needed at least two minutes to catch my breath. For my first 8 years in office, this fear confronted me each time I ascended the marble stairs of the State Capitol Building.

In March of 2003, I woke to numbness and tingling in my arm. An immediate visit to the doctor revealed I was suffering from obesity induced diabetes. My physician then said the words that opened my eyes forever, "If you don't make some changes, you're in the last decade of your life." Devastated by the news and angry at myself, I was forced to seriously reconsider the way I had been living.

First, some things had to go. Potato chips gone, double cheeseburgers gone, refined sugars gone, sitting on the couch finishing off what's left of Sunday's casserole right before nap time … gone! Taking personal responsibility for your health is the key and I hadn't been doing a very good job of being responsible for myself. There was always an excuse. I'm too busy, I have other responsibilities, I can't eat healthy on the go, and I can't find time to exercise. When I realized I might not live to meet my grandchildren, I knew it was time for the excuses to go.

With help from my doctor, support from my family, and a personal attitude change I lost over 110 lbs. in a little over a year. People always ask, "Alright, what's the secret? What diet pill did you take? What surgery did you have?" My answer's always the same; the secret is good old fashioned hard work. I exercise everyday and I don't put harmful foods into my body. I didn't find time to exercise and eat right, I made time. Now, my diagnosis of Type II diabetes … gone! It's as though I never had the disease. It was up to me to make the changes and I did.

Unfortunately too many Americans are still suffering. Currently diabetes threatens the lives of over 30 million people in our nation. Poor personal choices come at a great cost, the cost of health insurance, the cost of life, the cost of a family member or loved one. But if I can make the change, anyone can. It's time for America to put down the junk food, put on the sweatpants and toss excuses in the garbage instead of our health.

Despite the significant health risk attributable to diabetes, many Americans don't regard it as a serious threat. Dr. Bortz is a medical professional who is sounding the alarm about the dangers and astronomical costs of this disease. Through his affiliation with the Diabetes Research and Wellness Foundation, his many books, and his more than 150 scientific articles, Dr. Bortz has created a detailed picture of how our nation has fallen into poor health and opens our eyes to what we can do to reverse this trend.

Dr. Bortz's "gold standard" for the medical care of diabetes patients is a prescription for success. By focusing on personal responsibility and lifestyle change instead of costly medical treatment, diabetes patients can take on their illness and take control of their lives. Through adopting a healthy lifestyle Dr. Bortz shows us how to restore our "health wealth account" rather than depleting it.

A living example of his ideas, Dr. Bortz has run a marathon every year for the past 35 years. Not long ago I would have thought something like that was impossible for a person like me. How wrong I was! Inspired by my own weight loss I decided to go for it, and in April of 2005, I completed the Little Rock Marathon. Crossing that finish line was like crossing into a new world of possibilities. You can do it too, but you've got to start today. This book will change your attitude about diabetes and weight loss, but only you can change your life.

1

Diabetes Flashpoint

The roof is on fire.

Smoke billows, sirens sound. The wind howls, red lights flash, sparks fly, flames lick at the bedpost, and you sleep.

You don't hear all the commotion from your neighbor's house. Their house is on fire too. The entire neighborhood is on fire: an awful pandemic called diabetes is sweeping the entire globe. The world is on fire with diabetes, and most people—even many who already have this debilitating disease—ignore it. They do so at their peril.

Just a few years ago, in the United States there were fewer than one million diagnosed cases of diabetes. Today there are twenty million, and by 2030 there will be thirty million. A million new cases are diagnosed every year. On average the diagnosis of diabetes shortens a person's life by 15 years. Twenty million cases times 15 years equal 300 million years of life that will be lost by today's diabetics—a lot of time! Like the rumbles before a volcanic eruption, we recognize that the long interval between the onset of the disease and the occurence of its catastrophic complications will certainly shorten lives.

Bad, Really Bad

Go to a dictionary and look up the words horrible, ugly, painful, expensive, selfish, cruel, ferocious, relentless, and fearful. Each of these words describes diabetes. There is nothing good to be said about it, except if you get it, you darn well better take extra good care of yourself or these grim adjectives will describe your life.

This book will characterize diabetes in the worst, most vitriolic terms; the disease deserves it. It is truly horrible. Every single case is a disaster, but the tragedy is that the number of individual cases is going through the roof. A hundred years ago diabetes was a rare entry on death certificates. Now it is the fifth leading cause of death in the United States. Projecting its increased rise on the list of causes of death, from "rare" a few years ago to numbers 8, 7, 6, and now 5, we can objectively project that very soon it may be the number one killer—certainly a dubious distinction.

People can prevent themselves from getting diabetes and I'm hoping this book will help do just that. If that's your goal, make sure you read Chapters Three, Five and Six. If you already have diabetes and desire ways to effectively manage the disease, then Chapter Four, Five and Six are must-reads.

Silent Killer

Diabetes smolders before it erupts into flame. Usually at first it consumes its victims slowly, almost imperceptibly. It may start with a slight tinge and be followed with first, second, and third-degree burns. And then, even worse: blindness, kidney failure, stroke, or heart attack may follow. At the first sign of the disease's presence, immediate and meticulous care must be taken to guard against these ravages. If not, this deadly killer diabetes will consume its next victim.

At the time of their diagnosis, half of those millions suffering from Type 2 diabetes already have serious complications. By progressive singeing, the disease may silently do damage to the body's blood vessels, eyes, kidneys, and nerves. A long interval between the disease's onset and awareness of it can be a disaster.

It is estimated there may be as many people with unrecognized diabetes as there are who know of their condition. Occasionally a person develops a big-time problem such as coma without prior awareness of his diabetic condition. But more commonly, diabetes is a stealth disease in which its damage is done silently. This is why our health "fire alarms" must be set at a very low threshold of danger. In other words, the disease should be diagnosed as soon as possible. Just how long it takes to progress from its early pre-awareness smoldering to the full-fledged five alarm fire is currently a subject of intense scientific research. This book is intended to be a siren, an insistent screech intended to waken the world to this colossal threat.

Bad News, Good News

Diabetes is a killer, but even worse is this disease's tendency to torture before it kills. Millions of life years are ravaged by the many and various complications diabetes provokes. It is a leading cause of blindness in the United States, a major cause of heart attack and stroke, as well as a leading cause of kidney failure—all conditions which immensely diminish quality of life.

In my book, *We Live Too Short and Die Too Long*, I explored the important issue of quality of life. While how long we live is important, how we die may be even more important. If I were to name the worst feature of diabetes, I would say the tendency to induce dependency. Most of us value quality over quantity, so how many years of bad-quality life would you trade for one really good year? Are five years of blindness or 10 years of dialysis or 15 years with bilateral amputations a fair trade for one year of good life? The academics even have a code for this quandary: "quality adjusted life years." These scenarios are constructed in order to place a numerical value on life quality. The good news of course, is that when caught in time and expert care is taken to alter its course, diabetes is manageable and its complications may be avoided.

The Obesity Link

There is an even bigger epidemic than diabetes upon us—obesity. Obesity is defined as excessive accumulation of body fat in proportion to body size. It is known that obesity predisposes individuals to a variety of problems—diabetes, hypertension, stroke, arthritis, and heart disease, as well as the psychological and social stigma that accompanies it. Obesity and the conditions associated with it are among the leading causes of illness and premature death around the world.

Predictors of Diabetes

Obesity is determined by a measure of the body mass index (BMI), a system to compare weight regardless of body type. The BMI is determined by dividing the body weight in kilograms by the body height in meters squared. To determine your body mass, see Figure 24 in Appendix B. Using BMI, risk can be gauged for the development of various illnesses—such as diabetes, hypertension, and heart disease. Individuals with a normal weight have low incidence of these conditions, while those rated as overweight have an increased risk. An obese rating means one has a significant risk for these diseases. Raising the BMI unit by just one point increases the risk of diabetes by 13%.

BODY MASS INDEX (BMI)

Normal	18.5–24.9
Overweight	25–29.9
Obese	30–34.9
Extremely obese	40 or greater

Another measure which may be predictive of disease conditions is the distribution of body fat. In the apple shape fat accumulates in the abdomen; versus the pear shape, where fat accumulates in the hips. Individuals with a waist measurement greater than 40 inches (102cm) for men and greater than 35 inches (88 cm) for women have an increased risk of heart disease, diabetes,

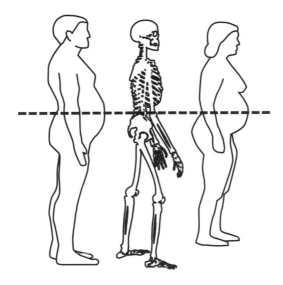

Figure 1. **Accurate Measurement of Waist Circumference**

(Abdominal Circumference in Adults)

stroke, and high blood pressure. (See Figure 1 to accurately measure waist circumference.)

Obesity is an open invitation to diabetes. No wonder it is so central to the origin of the blaze.

Globesity

A recent issue of *National Geographic* had a cover story about the absolutely unprecedented spike in the number of fat people in the world. Worldwide, there are now one billion overweight people—a doubling in 20 years. In China, between the years of 1989 and 1997, the number of people who were overweight doubled in women and tripled in men. In Singapore, a tiny country that by its size is super-vigilant to threats, does not promote children in school if their weight exceeds a standard value. In Africa, 3% of children are overweight, whereas 0.7% are underweight. The future is grim there, too. Europe is also focusing on fighting this epidemic by regulating fast food activities aimed at children.

Television specials, life insurers, news services, budget constructers of all types fret about this spreading epidemic. Furniture designers, barbers and beauticians, politicians, undertakers, airlines, nurses all face new problems with their customers' added heft. The seats in Yankee Stadium have been widened from 19 to 22 inches.

The Goliath Casket Company specializes in wide bodies. Recently, they created what might be the largest casket ever built, a seven foot, 84 inch, wide box built for a 900-pound Alaskan man. It was shipped by barge.

Most really big people can fit into a 52 inch coffin, which is as big as a double bed. In the 1990s, the largest casket was 38 inches in width, but demand has spurred a 48 inch version, which was then subsequently expanded to 52 inch.

Goliath's sales go up 20% per year. They sold 600 caskets last year, which is only a small fraction of all the oversize caskets sold in the United States. It is estimated that nationwide, 300 oversized caskets are sold per day; 15 years ago it was only two or three per day. Sometimes things go wrong: forklifts break, support stands buckle, doors are too narrow. Sometimes two gravesites are necessary to accommodate wider caskets.

The crematorium business is on alert as well. An obese corpse can generate twenty times the heat as a slim one during cremation, leading to concern about a meltdown of the oven.

The diabetes pandemic is mainly caused by the surge in world fat. Fat is the fuel feeding the flame. To douse the diabetes inferno, we must reduce globesity.

Forget Global Warming
Think Global Diabetes Wildfire

It's not just an American problem; it's happening everywhere. Worldwide in 2005 there were 171 million people with diabetes. By 2030, this figure is expected to double to 366 million. Globally there are 3.2 million deaths attributed to diabetes per year. This is probably a conservative estimate because frequently diabetes is not listed on the death certificate. Eight thousand seven hundred deaths a day, six deaths a minute are caused by diabetes. By 2030, India will have 62 million citizens with diabetes. That is equal to the entire population of Great Britain or France!

And, as we discussed, this accounting of the diabetes epidemic does not include the millions who are undiagnosed. While in developed countries most victims are over 65, in developing countries diabetes is striking a younger generation. No nation is immune or is safe from this deadly disease's awful reach.

Rapid Onset Diabetes

By surveying the different guises the disease adopts in young and old people, one can gain a more complete understanding of its dangers. One hundred years ago there was only one type of diabetes for both young and old and it had something to do with sweet urine. Now we look back and wonder how the experts of those days could have been so uninformed, not to know that young and old are very different. Around 1975 enough different lines of evidence converged to indicate that the centuries' old effort to lump all diabetes into a single category was wrong; Types 1 and 2—fast and slow diabetes—are now official. They are securely and separately identified. Categorically unique in causation and treatment, Types 1 and 2 are easily differentiated as well by their times of origin. Type 1 is kids, juvenile diabetes. Type 2 is adults, adult-onset diabetes, and that is that ... or so it seemed.

It is generally accepted that Type 1 occurs as a direct byproduct of the destruction of the beta cells of the pancreas. The origin of this destructive process is probably an offending antigen, possibly a virus. The body tries to counter such an attack by producing antibodies, which erroneously attack the beta cells, which produce insulin and related enzymes. These autoantibodies are detectable in the blood of most children with Type 1.

Patients with Type 1 are also prone to the development of other auto-immune diseases such as thyroid disease, adrenal gland insufficiency, sprue, and pernicious anemia. This association strengthens the auto-immune theory for the fundamental cause of Type 1 diabetes.

The disease is rapid and aggressive in infants and children. Within two to four weeks of its initial symptoms of frequent thirst and urination, fatigue and hunger, the diagnosis is established. Although Type 1 is found much more commonly in young people, it may even occur in the eighth and ninth decades of life.

Resistance to Insulin

Type 2 diabetes presents entirely different circumstances. Lack of insulin is not the problem: Resistance to insulin's action by the body's tissues is. What is the function of insulin? The complete answer to this simple question fills textbooks, but the short response is that it facilitates the movement of the blood sugar from the outside of the cells to the inside. Insulin is a key, which when inserted opens up the cell membranes so that sugar can enter, where it is burned as the body's main fuel. Insulin is necessary for all cells to use sugar. The muscles—most importantly; and the liver, the heart, and the brain—as well as every one of our body's 10 trillion cells, need insulin to fit into the lock so sugar may enter.

What causes this insensitivity, resistance to insulin? Two prime candidates appear: abdominal fat and physical inactivity. Forty years ago, Professor Philip J. Randall of the John Radcliffe Hospital in Oxford, England proposed that the main mechanism by which insulin resistance occurs is an imbalance between the body's use of fat and carbohydrate.

The connection between obesity and Type 2 diabetes (diabesity—a term coined by C. Everett Keep's "Shape Up America Program") is well established. Occasionally, however, an older person without obvious obesity can also suffer from Type 2 diabetes. One explanation for this seeming inconsistency is that obesity comes in different shapes: apples and pears. As previously mentioned,

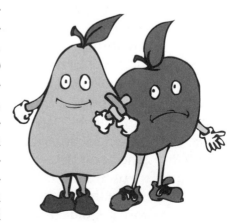

Figure 2.

apple obesity applies to those persons whose excess fat is distributed around the midriff. Pear-shaped obesity refers to those persons whose fat lies principally in their hips and buttocks.

Fascinating research indicates that these different types of obesity have different metabolic patterns. The apple form is more malevolent than the pear. So it is possible that some adults with an apple pattern of fat deposition may lead to Type 2 without being generally labeled as obese according to weight/ height tables. Some feel that waist size is a more accurate predictor of eventual diabetes than weight or BMI.

The shocking new story of kids with diabetes is the evil entry of Type 2 into their age range. This phenomenon is so abrupt and unexpected that there are yet to be any statistics which capture its invasion into a time of life where it doesn't belong. Not that there is a proper time and place for this awful disease, yet somehow it is slightly easier to rationalize an adult rather than a child succumbing to a lifestyle disease characterized by physical inactivity and obesity.

Early Lessons

Fifty years ago, when I was in medical school at the University of Pennsylvania, diabetes was already an important disease that occupied a substantial spot in our curriculum and experience on the wards. We learned that it was an extremely serious illness with a high mortality rate. Most of its victims were young, in their teens and twenties. Once diagnosed, these young persons were treated with insulin, which was still fairly early in its clinical application having been first discovered as a therapy in 1922.

Insulin's formulation was primitive and our use of it was equally crude. As a result, the diabetic control of these young persons was poor, with frequent excursions of their blood sugar levels from very high to very low. Both of these extremes provoked trips to the emergency room, and the seesaw of adequate treatment was rarely balanced. For these reasons we employed the term "brittle diabetes" to describe the erratic nature of our patients' illness.

Rarely did we see older patients with high blood sugar. And we reserved the term "adult-onset diabetes" for them because it was a very different proposition. Instead of the other aggressive, nasty nature of the juvenile with the disease, the suffering older person rarely got into the pickles the younger ones did. Usually its onset was gradual and the severe acute side effects such as too low or too high blood sugar levels were missing, In short, the adults with diabetes were uninteresting to us young doctors-to-be. The older had difficulties, but much later in life. Type 2 was a disease of aging and a seeming minor urgency.

In the past few years, the picture has totally changed. Now almost all new cases of diabetes are of the adult-onset variety, but their onset is not confined to older folks. Now the pediatricians are seeing adult-onset diabetes in increasing numbers, even in their age group. We don't have figures, yet what I hear from the pediatricians I know is that the commonest pattern in their practices is now Type 2. This is a sad commentary on our culture because we know that these burdened kids didn't have to get diabetes. Our culture, not a virus, gave it to them.

Our Young People Are in Grave Danger

Dr. Francine R. Kaufman, esteemed pediatric endocrinologist at UCLA, relates some vignettes about this circumstance in her wonderful book *Diabesity*.

Dr. Kaufman tells of being called to see a 13-year-old African-American girl in the emergency room because her blood sugar was four times the normal level. The ER doctor had called Kaufman in to consult because of the girl's alarming blood test result. But despite her sky-high blood sugar, the girl appeared okay, and was in fact eating fries and drinking soda at the time the call was made. The girl was 5 feet 3 inches tall and weighed 267 pounds. A careful history taking revealed that for a year the girl did have typical symptoms of frequent thirst and urination, which clearly had not provoked any weight loss. Her grandmother had had diabetes for 30 years, having had a foot amputated and a paralyzing stroke. The older woman acknowledged that she had been derelict about her own care, despite full knowledge of her diagnosis. "Taking insulin makes me feel bad." Now she was reaping the complications that resulted from this abdication.

The circumstances of the granddaughter are now commonplace. What once was a rare condition is now the rule. In 1997 a representative committee of the American Diabetes Association and the World Health Organization recommended that the term "adult-onset diabetes" be abandoned and renamed Type 2 (a new term) since the disease was being found in all age groups.

While diabetes shows no gender preference, it does target certain population groups: African-Americans, Hispanics, American Indians, and Pacific Islanders appear to be more susceptible. This reality poses particular hazard to those host countries from which these persons emigrated because once they become westernized and inactive, which means fat, their number of people getting the disease is sure to climb.

Since Type 2 has only recently been recognized in young people, it is not possible to forecast what their futures hold. A study of Canadian Indian children is not reassuring. Dr. Heather Dean recently looked at the records of children with Type 2 diabetes ages 18 to 23 that suffered from Type 2 for at least 10 years. She found that 9% had died, and another 6% were on renal dialysis—a terrible story.

Our Broken Health Care System

One of the largely unacknowledged reasons behind the spreading inferno called diabetes is that our "fire department" is ill-trained and equipped for the emergency. Like a giant intensive care unit, the medical care system is designed to respond to acute conditions often due to a singular external cause such as injury or infection or even malignancy. But diabetes does not fit into that category of conditions in which the medical system excels. It is largely a lifestyle-caused disease for which the technological fixes of the medical system are insufficient.

Not that medicine doesn't try to extinguish diabetes through technology, in the implicit hope that this may retard the blaze. It is estimated there will be 200,000 stomach stapling procedures performed this year—at $30,000 a pop. But with almost 200 million overweight persons in America alone, of whom at least 40 million already have diabetes or are on their way to getting it, the stomach stapling doctors are going to have to pick up their pace.

The point is that health care professionals are not adequately dealing with this epidemic. And if you're not part of the solution, you must be part of the problem. The fire department gets paid to put flames out. They wait until the blaze starts and then scramble to deal with the situation. With diabetes, this strategy is not working.

In the World Health Organization's regular survey of global health, the United States gets first place in just one category: cost. In all other categories we rank far down the list. Evaluating the *overall* health of each country, WHO ranks the United States as 37th—behind many countries with far less prosperity than our own.

Later in the book we will take a deeper look at the shameful performance of the United States health care system in confronting the diabetes inferno. In my view, the American public has mistakenly been sold a viewpoint that our medical profession can handle all blazes—from backyard grass fires to full-blown six alarm blazes. Famed economist and Nobel Laureate Gary Becker recently observed that Americans don't heed the many warnings to their health because of a misplaced faith in science to solve all problems.

Type 2 Flares Up

Diabetes is not new. It has been around a long time, initially as scattered sad cases that invariably died soon after being diagnosed. With the 1922 introduction of insulin as a treatment, individuals with Type 1 diabetes started to live.

In the past 15 years there has been a rapid spike of incidence of Type 2 diabetes and this distressing trend shows no signs of letting up. The accompanying diabetes maps provided by the Centers for Disease Control illustrate how rapidly this disease is engulfing our nation.

As disturbing as the diabetes mapping is, the overweight/obesity mapping is even worse. Pretty soon, the whole world will be up in flames. The tables in Figure 4 represent the surge in our BMIs at all ages.

Figure 3. **Estimates of Diagnosed Diabetes Among Adults**

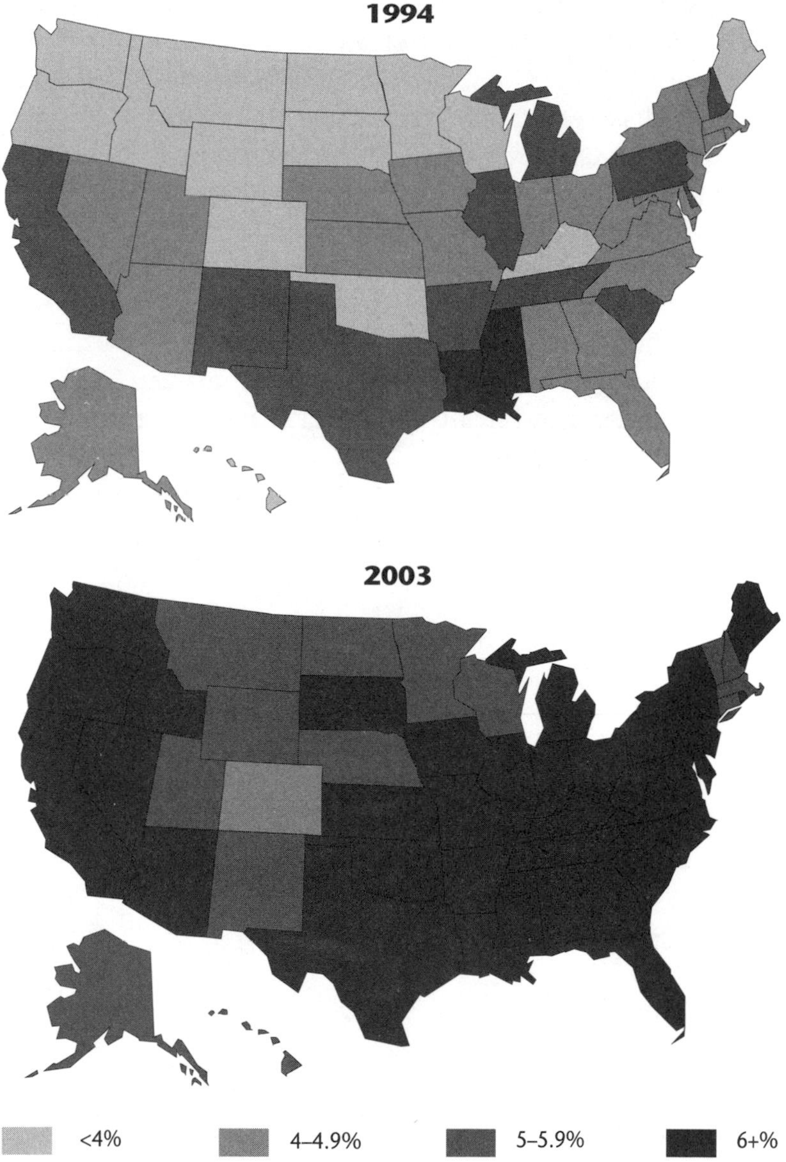

1994

2003

<4%   4–4.9%   5–5.9%   6+%

Humanity Destroying Itself

Although the genus Homo has been around for a few million years this isn't a long time on a cosmic time scale. Ninety-nine percent of all species that have ever lived are now extinct; they came and went leaving few traces to remember their passing. The dinosaurs and the millions of other extinct earthly creatures who populated our planet have no archivists to record their decline and fall. The fact that human beings have survived many prior disasters is no guarantee that new technologies won't cause our extinction. The muddle-through argument is not convincing. We are now doing things that we have never done before.

Pulitzer-Prize-winning Jared Diamond's new book *Collapse* takes an encyclopedic look at the features which characterize some of the famous and not-so-famous fallen civilizations. The Australian Aborigines, the Vikings, the American Indians, the Mayans, the Easter and Pitcairn Islanders each reveal their extinction trajectories and causes.

Having closely studied these collapses, Diamond writes "much more likely than a doomsday scenario for human extinction is one deriving from lower living standards which might assume the form of worldwide disease or wars."

Figure 4. **Surge of BMI Rates**

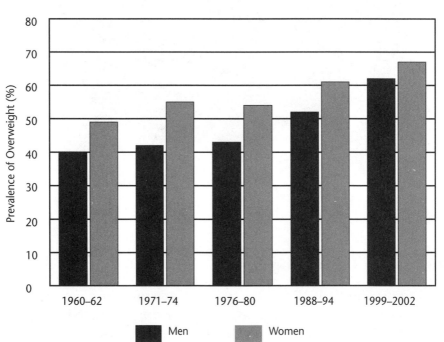

He warns against false alarms and not responding to every blip on the radar screen. Diamond observes that the fall of the Roman Empire in 476 "was due not to invading tribes but to social and value decay within the citizenry." He concludes by suggesting that our collapse would more likely occur because of "conditions that we generate ourselves rather than from a meteor or a tidal wave."

This projection makes much sense. The current largest threat to the survival of the human race arises from the absolutely unique collision between two components of humanity: biology and capitalism. The diabesity threat is the direct result of this violent clash. Two primal forces at the core of our existence are in conflict. A red alert sounds.

Seize Our Destiny

Our body's biology is the evolutionary byproduct of millions of years of trial and error. The human body's fuel tanks are fat. They

Surge of BMI Rates (Continued)

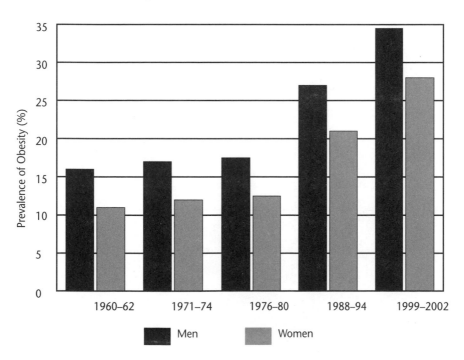

see us through lean times. And under normal conditions, these tanks serve us admirably. But when they are over-filled, they present a potential for disaster. Obesity, accompanied by abdication of our primitive vigorous physical activity patterns, sets the stage for disaster.

P I (Physical Inactivity) + O (Overweight) = D (Diabetes).

The Serenity Prayer wonderfully encourages us to change what we can, accept what we must, but, to *know the difference.* If mankind's destiny is predetermined by Fate, by forces beyond our reach, we're cooked. But if our future is truly ours to construct, then we better get busy fixing it.

2

The History and Causes of Diabetes

For centuries, the best physicians have been studying people suffering from diabetes. These patients have been wildly diverse: some were men, some were women, some young, some old. Some had trouble with their heart, others with their legs, and still others with their sex lives. Some patients were fat, others were thin. Some died as soon as they caught the disease; others lived a long time with it. Some were pregnant. Some were dark, some were light.

The one common feature in all of this confusion is that these people passed a lot of urine. But aside from this common symptom, physicians over the years asked themselves, "How can I better understand and treat this disease?"

Such was the sorry state of knowledge about diabetes for even the best physicians until just a few years ago. Even though diabetes has been noted since the dawn of recorded history, confusion has reigned.

Digging Deep

Every fire inquiry starts with an analysis of the setting and the timeline. Any medical examination starts with a history of the illness. What were the first clues that something was amiss? When did they occur? What were the predisposing circumstances? Any family history of the disease?

When you dig back into the history of diabetes it turns out that you need a long-handled shovel to dig deep enough to capture all the fascinating details of its occurrence. And further, it turns out that these inquiries into the ancient origins of diabetes have direct relevance to the alarming health emergency we now face.

Diabetes' First Diagnosticians

Ancient Hindu scriptures include the observation that ants and flies had a particular attraction to the urine of persons dying of a mysterious, deadly disease. These were the first diagnosticians of what we now know as diabetes.

An Egyptian papyrus from 1552 B.C. described a patient with symptoms typical of diabetes. In 250 B.C., Apollonius of Memphis coined the word "diabetes" from a Greek word meaning siphon— indicating that such persons produced excessive amounts of urine. At that time, children who were affected by the syndrome were recognized as having an abrupt, rapidly fatal course—Type 1 diabetes, while older persons experienced a slower progress that featured dreadful complications—later called Type 2 diabetes. Another Greek word *mellitus,* meaning honey, was appended to diabetes. This recognized the relation of sugar to the disease.

In 150 A.D., Aretaeus, the Cappadocian described diabetes as being more common in women and associated with the melting of flesh into urine. Life with Type 1 diabetes was short and death was speedy. Life was disgusting and thirst unquenchable, like scorched by fire.

The Hindus are credited with the first recognition of the association of Type 2 diabetes with obesity. And in 1000 A.D., Greek physicians prescribed

SYMPTOMS OF DIABETES
Fatigue
Extreme thirst
Frequent urination
Unexplained weight loss
Blurred vision
Non-healing wounds

exercise, preferably on horseback, as a treatment to establish moderate friction, which was intended to alleviate excess urination.

The importance of the pancreas as the source of insulin was not even considered until 1788 when Thomas Cawley recorded the scarred distortion of this gland in a person who had died from a condition resembling diabetes. In 1798, John Rollo, a physician in Britain, was the first to demonstrate high levels of sugar in the urine and blood of persons with *diabetes mellitus*. He also noted the increased amounts of sugar in the urine after a starchy diet and subsequently advised a high protein diet.

Claude Bernard, a French physician of historic significance, grew closer to a fuller understanding. In the mid-1800s, his experiments led him to conclude that the liver was the main culprit in diabetes by making too much sugar out of the starch and glycogen, which the liver stores.

A series of minor discoveries led to the conclusion that a specific type of cell within the pancreas, the beta cell, was the manufacturing unit of insulin. These beta cells, in turn, are aggregated into groups called the islets of Langerhans. In the pancreas there are perhaps 3 million islets. German medical student Paul Langerhans, described them in 1869, but failed to grasp their significance. Langerhans did, however, recognize that whatever these islands of cells made was most likely being directly circulated in the blood. In 1870, the French physician, A. Bouchardet noticed the disappearance of sugar from the urine of his diabetic patients during the rationing occasioned by the German siege in the Franco-German War.

Finally, two German physicians Joseph von Mering and Oscar Minkowski—who shared an interest in digestion—conducted an important, historic experiment. In 1889, they surgically removed a dog's pancreas to observe the effects on the animal's digestion. The next day the dog's caretaker bitterly complained that this previously-housebroken animal was uncontrollably urinating and soiling the room. The genie was out of the bottle: somehow the pancreas was making something which controlled the level of blood sugar, and as blood sugar levels rose, it prompted a profuse outpouring of urine as a direct result.

Eureka!

On May 15, 1921, a young Canadian physician, Frederick Banting, awoke with a startling idea. He had just recently attended a lecture by Dr. Moses Barron in which Barron described how the changes in the pancreas after tying its drainage tubes were similar to those pancreatic changes caused by tubes plugged up by gallstones. Banting arose and wrote in his notebook, "Ligate the pancreatic duct. Wait six to eight weeks for degeneration. Remove the residue and extract." This moment was the genesis of our use of insulin.

Banting impatiently awaited the return from Scotland of his boss, Dr. J.J.R. Macleod, director of the physiology laboratory at the University of Toronto. Eventually, Macleod provided Banting with a lab, ten dogs, and a young assistant, Charles H. Best.

Banting and Best set to work. On July 27, 1921, eight teaspoonfuls of a pancreatic extract of a dog whose tube had been previously tied off were injected into the vein of another dog, who was diabetic after the removal of its pancreas. The blood sugar of the diabetic dog fell from 200 to 110 within two hours! A second dog was kept alive for 70 days using the revolutionary extract. This was the first time in history when insulin had been given successfully to living animals.

Success brought problems: the extracts were still too crude and caused toxicity and sepsis at the point of injection. To address this problem, chemist J. B. Collip joined the group. With his help, the extracts were progressively refined and purified.

With little public reaction, this exciting story was first reported at a medical meeting, in New Haven, CT in December 1921, followed by a presentation to the Association of American Physicians in May 1922.

On July 11, 1922, seven patients with diabetes in Toronto General Hospital were treated with injection of the pancreas extract. The first was Leonard Thompson, a 14-year-old boy weighing just 65 pounds. Leonard's blood sugars promptly fell. The clinical usefulness of insulin was proven!

The first official publication of the results was in the *Canadian Medical Association Journal* in 1922 under the title "Pancreatic Extracts in Treatment of Diabetes Mellitus." This breakthrough was immediately acclaimed. The Nobel Prize was awarded to Macleod and Banting in 1923. Macleod split his award with Collip, Banting split his with Best.

The dark ages of diabetes—years of total ignorance, fear, pain, and ignoble death—began to recede before the lightening of shadows provided by knowledge. However, much work remains to be done.

Confusing Types 1 and 2

Although diabetes has been around for a long time, not until recently was any differentiation made between Type 1 from 2. Out of curiosity, I took out my *Cecil and Loeb,* the standard textbook of medicine from my medical student days. It was interesting to reread the chapter on diabetes. In 1955, there was still ignorance and confusion, with no differentiation as to types of diabetes. The discovery of this differentiation had vast implications, as we shall see.

Just yesterday, I discovered another wonderful old resource in the far corner of my library. Dr. Shields Warren was the pathologist for Elliott Joslin at the Deaconess Hospital shortly after insulin was discovered. Dr. Warren's 1930 book is entitled *The Pathology of Diabetes Mellitus,* which at the time was *the* definitive text on the topic.

Warren records meticulous studies of the pancreas and other tissues of persons with diabetes. It is intriguing to see the confusions that Dr. Warren faced in 1930 trying to make sense out of the lack of consistency in the microscopic slides of the patients studied. What he saw through the microscope in most of the young subjects was evidence of inflammation of the beta cells, an indication of an attack on the insulin-producing cells in the pancreas, which we now know signifies Type 1 diabetes. In contrast, most of his older patients had fat deposits in the beta cells, as well as everywhere else—Type 2 diabetes. All of his adult patients showed evidence of advanced arteriosclerosis. Many of the specimens showed clear evidence that the pancreas was in the active business of trying to heal itself from some unknown injury. The body's ceaseless efforts to counteract the effects of physical inactivity and obesity causes pancreatic stress. The islet cells become unhappy as a result.

Much of Dr. Warren's confusion can now be explained by the different types of diabetes we know about today.

No One Description Fits All

Each form of diabetes is different in causation, clinical course, and treatment. No single description makes sense.

It was not until 1957 that Solomon Berson and Rosalynn Yalow detected and measured minute amounts of insulin in the blood. At last, this newfound capacity confirmed the suspicion that diabetes mellitus was really two different forms of diabetes. Type 1 (insulin-dependent diabetes or juvenile diabetes) results from an insulin deficiency in which no insulin is found. In Type 2 diabetes (insulin- resistant diabetes or non-insulin dependent diabetes or adult-onset diabetes), insulin is present, in some cases in elevated amounts, but the insulin produced by the body is somehow ineffective.

Types 1 and 2 diabetes both result in high levels of blood sugar. Importantly, they also share common complications, due to the diversion of these high sugar levels into other chemical compounds. These compounds silently smolder, damaging blood vessels throughout the body. The result can be kidney disease, heart disease, blindness, amputation and nerve damage.

Where There's Smoke, There's Fire

Type 2 diabetes doesn't happen all of a sudden. Its onset happens slowly over a period of time. A sequence of subtle changes silently occurs, which after a number of years leads to the diagnosis of diabetes.

The early phases of diabetes diagnosis and care can be extremely confusing. I recall from my personal practice several instances when I reported to patients that our tests showed their blood sugar levels were clearly elevated. This disclosure is life-altering. However, several times, a repeat check up in a month revealed that these patients' blood sugar was back in the normal range. I suspect this sort of mixed-signals caused my patients to wonder about my competence.

What was happening in the above cases is called a "diabetic honeymoon" in which the initial diagnosis seems to have been mistaken. Unfortunately, after several more months the honeymoon ends, and the diabetes is permanently in place.

This phenomenon of temporary recovery is generally thought to be due to the pancreas' beta cells somehow becoming active again, and making enough insulin to control sugar levels. Maybe the cells were temporarily "shocked" by high levels of blood sugar or blood fat. This lull in the fire unfortunately is short-lived and the process then resumes its evil course.

Normally there is a very specific relationship between the blood sugar level and insulin release. Diabetes represents an uncoupling between the two, and early in the progression from the normal to the full blown state of diabetes strange disjunctions such as the honeymoon offer evidence of the body's effort to compensate for the new challenges being confronted.

The Earliest Possible Diagnosis

The level of blood sugar rises after a meal and falls after insulin kicks in as seen in Figure 5. The level of the blood sugar measured first thing in the morning (FBS) after an overnight fast has been the gold standard for "normalcy." For almost all doctors the level of the FBS is the most commonly used measurement tool to diagnose diabetes.

Importantly, the diabetes experts have progressively lowered the level of accepted normalcy, trying to make the diagnosis at the earliest possible moment so that the ominous, early smoke signals can be heeded.

Now the consensus is that if the FBS is 126 or above, the diagnosis is made. But what if it is 115 or 105 or 95? If we are intent on providing the earliest diagnosis, is it possible that these marginal blood sugar levels might contain warning information?

DIAGNOSTIC CRITERIA FOR DIABETES

Fasting blood sugar $\geq$ 126 mg/dl (7.0 mmol/l)

Blood sugar $\geq$ 200 mg/dl (11.1 mmol/l) two hours after drinking a 75g glucose dissolved in water, during a glucose tolerance test

---

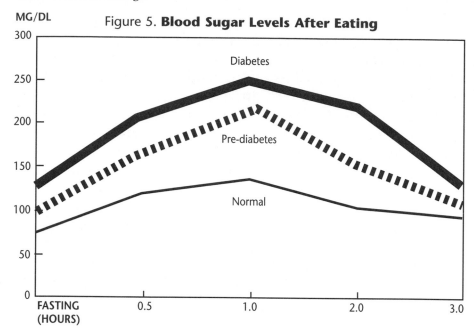

MG/DL
Figure 5. **Blood Sugar Levels After Eating**

Diabetes

Pre-diabetes

Normal

300

250

200

150

100

50

0

FASTING
(HOURS)   0.5   1.0   2.0   3.0

An Empty Gas Tank and a Heavy Load

A person suffering from Type 1 is like a car with a big hole in the fuel tank. Think of insulin as fuel. In order for the Type 1 car to get anywhere, it requires a constant supply of fuel. In contrast, the Type 2 car starts out with a non-leaking full tank, but the poor car with only 4 cylinders is dragging a heavy trailer of cinder blocks. For the Type 2 car to get anywhere, it strains, laboring in low gear, it gets terrible mileage, and eventually it burns out its engine and brakes. Along the way, the unfit Type 2 can help itself by unhitching its burdensome trailer—that is, if too much wear and tear has not already occurred. If the load is not removed then, like Type 1, with the hole in the tank, Type 2 will need insulin from outside.

Fast Diabetes

I think of Type 1 as "Fast Diabetes." To further use the analogy, this "fast" distinction of Type 1 from Type 2 is appropriate because Type 1 is due to the insulin-leaking fuel tank. It occurs abruptly and, without insulin treatment, it will kill abruptly. This was the typical story in young diabetics before 1922. Type 1 had an outside cause.

The leading candidate for the villainous cause of Type 1 diabetes is the body's own defense system. We've known for a long time that the body possesses an elaborate set of defenses designed to combat foreign proteins such as bacteria and viruses. These same sets of reactive antibodies are responsible for the rejection of skin grafts or for a transfusion reaction after mismatched blood. Doctors will occasionally note an increase in the incidence of cases of Type 1 after a viral epidemic. Measles, mumps, and polio, like virus, have been incriminated among possible offending agents. It seems the immune system erroneously produces antibodies that end up attacking and destroying the beta cells—yielding Type 1 diabetes. Or later in life, Type 1 can be the result of external factors. Inflammation of the pancreas—as in pancreatitis, or cancer when advanced—can cause enough destruction to lead to diabetes.

I will never forget my patient David Thompson, a freckled, red-headed 11-year-old kid who got smacked with diabetes. The intense first session with him and his mother was exhausting for all. For him, as for all juvenile diabetics, the psychosocial elements were much more important than the bare medical facts. Upon his diagnosis, he became "different" from the average kid he was just the day before.

David was wonderfully faithful in recording his urine sugar tests, and brought in his urine test diary on his monthly visits. I recalled juggling his NPH insulin and regular insulin schedules, eventually adopting a twice-a-day regimen. Even then, the reports were extremely erratic and punctuated by occasional insulin reactions, which fortunately were mild.

I recall David so specifically because he was such a wonderful boy with such promise. I gave him my best for the eight or nine years before he went off to college. I hope that my earnest efforts gave him a chance to pursue his future decades with knowledge, confidence, and health. No question that I personally felt challenged by this, David's lifetime challenge. Doing one's best in such cases may provide a physician with immense gratification, but that comes with the concern that the care is adequate to meet the complexities and uncertainties presented by juvenile diabetes.

The Four Stages of Type 1

The University of Colorado's Diabetes Study Group identifies four stages in the course of Type 1:

1. Development of antibodies with progressive defect in insulin secretion
2. Onset of clinical diabetes
3. Transient remission
4. Established diabetes complete with secondary complications

The duration of Stage 1 varies, from as short as a few weeks to 13 years. Younger children tend to have a more rapid transit through the stages. Stage 3, the remission phase, the "honeymoon" phenomenon noted above, occurs in an uncertain number of patients, but is thought to represent the beta cells' attempt to heal.

Twenty to forty percent of Type 1 patients younger than 20 years of age are first diagnosed at the time of crisis called ketoacidosis, a condition in which the body lacks insulin and as a result breaks down fat for energy. Ketones are acids which build up in the blood and can poison the body—a life-threatening situation. Before there was insulin, nearly all persons with Type 1 died from this complication.

Although Type 1 is seen in all racial groups, it is more common in Caucasians. Sex incidence is equal. Fifty percent of those who contract Type 1 are under 20 years old, hence the old term "juvenile diabetes." However, sadly, even older people can contract it.

Slow Diabetes

It is estimated that 340,000 persons have Type 1 diabetes. While 19,750,000 have Type 2, or 98.75% of the total 20 million diabetics. Even this high percentage of Type 2 is an underestimate as the obesity epidemic claims more victims of Type 2 each and every moment.

With Type 1, there is almost no latent period between its cause (destruction of the beta cells) and the abrupt appearance of its severe symptoms (thirst, increased urination, weight loss, and weakness). However, the initial events involved with Type 2 represent such an occult process that the dating of its first event is imprecise.

The mean age of Type 2 diagnosis is 56. Data from 2000 say the following have Type 2 diabetes: 2.2% of persons in their twenties and thirties, 9.7% of those in their forties and fifties, 18.3% of persons in their sixties and seventies. 25% of those over 80 have Type 2 diabetes..

RISK FACTORS FOR TYPE 2 DIABETES
Obesity
Sedentary lifestyle
Race/ethnicity (African Americans, American Indians, Asians, Pacific Islanders, and Hispanic Americans)
Gestational diabetes during pregnancy
Delivery of a larger than average-weight baby
Family history
Polycystic ovary syndrome
Peripheral vascular disease
High blood pressure
High cholesterol levels
Coronary heart disease

Believe it or not, beyond these numbers lie even more ominous figures. Data from the Centers for Disease Control (CDC) and the National Institutes of Health (NIH) indicate 41 million Americans have pre-diabetes.

Half of all the identified cases of diabetes are in people over 55 years of age. The question arises as to whether aging itself may cause diabetes. Looking at the statistics, you might assume that, as you age, you might expect to become diabetic. You might also assume that you'll get fatter and lose muscle. These commonly-observed attributions of the "aging process" are in most geriatric textbooks.

In 2000, 69.4% of persons over 60 were overweight. In 2010, this figure is projected to be 72.3%. For the large part of my professional career I have been committed to differentiating those changes that are naturally part of the aging process and those which are due to other agencies.

Physical Inactivity + Obesity (+ Aging?) = Type 2 Diabetes

I wrote a major paper in the *Journal of the American Medical Association* entitled "Disuse and Aging." I argued that many or most of the physical changes experienced by older persons are not in fact, due to the aging process. They are due to disuse, and thereby are potentially reversible and preventable. The diminished muscle strength, bone density, nerve reactivity, artery size, circulatory competence, etc. that are listed in geriatric textbooks as being results of the aging process are, in fact, due to a lack of physical activity.

Included in this long list of preventable, negative consequences of aging, is diabetes due to aging alone. Impaired glucose tolerance of older persons is reversible by a fitness program—as are almost all of the other supposed "age changes."

If a function can be improved, then by definition it cannot be aging, because as far as I know, no one has ever been able to halt the fall of the grains of sand in the hourglass of life. In other words, aging happens resolutely, immutably, but cannot be held accountable for all the grim imagery, including Type 2 diabetes, which some have been increasingly, but wrongly, labeling as just another facet of growing older.

We know that Type 2 diabetes doesn't happen all of a sudden. Students of diabetes have long recognized that the early phases of Type 2 diabetes diagnosis and care can be incredibly confusing. Type 2 diabetes is so slow that it can smolder for years before being discovered. But it is just this slowness that makes it so vicious: the entire body is being quietly cooked by the degenerative processes caused by high blood sugar levels.

The kind of diabetes that didn't interest us in medical school 50 years ago is now setting off the emergency fire alarms. The health care emergency is Type 2 diabetes.

The Delicate Relationship between Fats and Carbohydrates

The reciprocal relationship between the two main body fuels of fats and carbohydrates is finely tuned. This relationship prompts dozens of searching scientific explorations to this day, but the fundamental interplay of fat and carbohydrate is critical to the understanding of Type 2 diabetes and resistance to insulin's primary function.

When an animal starves (and thus lacks carbohydrate as fuel), it immediately switches to its energy storage tanks (which are fat). Eight hours after the start of a fast, such as an overnight typical pattern, the blood levels of the free fatty acids go up threefold, and they become the principal fuel.

The smart body recognizes this and immediately switches its furnace to burn an alternate fuel, fat. When a meal is eaten, the reverse occurs, which requires that carbohydrate be used preferentially. Fat reverts to its storage depository role. This reciprocal switching is constant. Ordinarily, the elaborate bio-chemical network succeeds with incredible effectiveness and efficiency. Even long periods of starvation can be tolerated by a person with not much disturbance to their body functions. In prehistoric times of feast and famine, this compensatory elegance was crucial to our survival.

A New Factor: Obesity

Enter an entirely new player in this scenario: obesity. The metabolic fuel mix of the obese person is altered because of the increased traffic in fat. Reciprocally, carbohydrate and sugar use by the muscles is reduced, leading to higher blood sugar levels. These elevated levels alert the pancreas to pump out more insulin in an effort to lower the blood sugar levels. If this over stimulation persists for too long they become exhausted and insulin deficiency occurs.

Obesity is hardly part of our Darwinian development. Our bodies are designed to function otherwise. It is a novelty, not only in human terms, but in animal life in general. Domestication breeds obesity, and it is now upon us big-time. Even our pet dogs and cats mirror their owners' epidemic pattern of obesity and diabetes. (25% are overweight.)

An Invitation to Diabetes

All the evidence isn't in yet, but we do know that obesity causes Type 2 diabetes as a consequence of maladaptations. The body is trying to fix something that is broken, but Mother Nature overdoes it.

But fat isn't the only villain. Lack of physical activity is a critical co-conspirator. In diabetic laboratory animals, there is evidence that exercise promotes glucose use even in the absence of insulin. Exercise has been shown to have strong positive effects on the way muscle cells use insulin.

One thing is clear: Obesity and lack of fitness are interdependent co-conspirators and are the causes of the Type 2 diabetes epidemic.

A Genetic Predisposition?

But isn't there a family predisposition to diabetes? There's certainly an increased family incidence of diabetes when one (40%) or two (80%) parents are overweight. Does the same story apply to diabetes?

Students of diabetes were licking their chops in anticipation when the Human Genome Project was being unveiled. The Magic Bullet, the Holy Grail of Science was going to be available on the Internet yielding solutions to hordes of vexing problems, including diabetes.

The suggestion of a hereditary component to diabetes was bolstered by observations of many instances within several members of a single-family, as well as the clear predisposition of certain racial groups to develop the disease. "The thrifty gene hypothesis" has gained favor, which seems to indicate why persons of aboriginal origin show a higher incidence of obesity and diabetes. This theory proposes that certain indigenous populations have inherited a tendency to gain weight as a result of evolutionary processes which allowed their ancestors to survive starvation pressures. But the fact that—until the Aborigines came into Alice Springs or the Pima Indians crossed the Rio Grande—these people did not get fat, suggests that genes are not the issue. These thrifty genes don't change during these trips, these people's lifestyles did.

The Human Genome Project yielded no one answer. It turns out that dozens of different genes are involved in the production of diabetes and obesity. A "quick fix" solution remains a fantasy.

Forget about Genes, Change Your Lifestyle

Hence the emphasis is on lifestyle intervention in combating the blaze, instead of awaiting the remote, if ever, arrival of a new set of genes which do not encourage Type 2.

Our biology works well when we let it. It trembles when it is burdened by too little physical activity and too much fat.

Diabetes and Pregnancy

A discussion of the types and causes of diabetes requires mention of another category entitled "gestational diabetes." This condition, basically a subtype of Type 2, is identified as diabetes occurring in a previously unsuspecting woman when she becomes pregnant. This occurs in 4% of pregnancies, 135,000 cases per year. Fortunately, with good attention to lifestyle, weight management and exercise, it can be adequately managed. Without such care, the pregnant woman with a newly discovered elevation in blood sugar is at risk for a whole set of complications for herself and her baby.

Syndrome X

So what do high blood sugar, high blood fats, apple-shaped obesity, high blood pressure, and insulin resistance have to do with one another? These diverse, seemingly unrelated conditions are found in combination in older people so commonly that they have been grouped into an odd and obscure term "Syndrome X" or the "Metabolic Syndrome." NIH estimates that 47 million adults have this combination. Sixty percent of obese women have it.

Grouping terms together sometimes helps to explain their connection. Insulin resistance has been suggested as the primary event causing all the others. However, scientists have yet to figure out how insulin resistance would lead to the other complications and components of Syndrome X.

Steve Blair of the Cooper Aerobics Institute in Dallas cleared up this confusion. By using the huge set of observations of their clinic attendees, Steve says that the inciting circumstance to Syndrome X is physical inactivity.

Sixty percent of his obese subjects had Syndrome X, while 5% of normal weight subjects had Syndrome X. Thirty minutes of moderate intensity exercise on most days of the week, similar to the generally advocated recommendations, offered a method to protect a person from Syndrome X. Steve's hypothesis makes sense. As people age, they become progressively less active and as they retire from life, life retires from them, sometimes in the form of Syndrome X.

Syndrome X is important because it contains many of the risk factors for cardiovascular disease, which is the principal cause of illness and death in adults, particularly older ones.

A Lesson We've Yet to Learn

A fascinating insight into the recentness of diabetes is provided by an article published in the *Archives of Internal Medicine* in November 1924. It was called "Diabetes Mellitus, a Contribution to its Epidemiology, Based Chiefly on Mortality Statistics." Its authors were Drs. Herman Emerson and Louise Carson of the Public Health School of Columbia University. This paper is a rendering of the causes of death for the City of New York for the years 1866 to 1922 (the year insulin was born). In 1866, there were 11 deaths recorded from diabetes out of a population of 770,000, four of these deaths were in people under 25 and five over 45. In 1923, there were 1,360 deaths of diabetes from a population of 5.4 million. Fifty-four of these deaths were of persons under 20 years of age, 1,213 over 45. The rate of deaths from diabetes was two per 100,000 in 1866, rising to 22 per 100,000 in 1922.

Fascinating too, were Emerson and Carson's data on the occupational histories of those who developed diabetes. It is interesting to note that the higher incidences of diabetes occurred in the occupations that did not require physical activity, as seen in Figure 6. The death rates from diabetes were negligible for laborers. However, there were 180 deaths per 100,000 for bartenders, the highest rate; 120 per 100,000 for clergyman, the next highest; 40 per 100,000 for physicians, and 52 per 100,000 for policemen.

Emerson and Carson report on the sugar consumption in New York City during the era, showing striking parallels in the increased incidence of diabetes and sugar consumption over the same time interval.

Accounting for this "enlarging cloud on the horizon," they concluded "Moderation in the use of food and sufficient exercise with the entire body to justify the food absorbed, are important rules of hygiene for other reasons beyond that of the relationship between obesity and diabetes, but if there were no other excuse

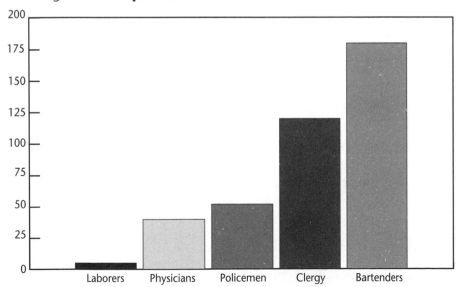

Figure 6. **Occupational Histories of Those with Diabetes**

for bringing the ancient teaching to people's attention, the greatly increased frequency of diabetes as a cause of sickness and death would alone seem to justify physicians and all those dealing with health and its protection in initiating and pursuing vigorously a campaign of information on the subject." This was 81 years ago!

Bushmen Lessons

I have forever been an amateur anthropologist. I figure that one of the most important fields of study for us mere mortals is the understanding of how we got to be who we are today. In pursuit of this major hobby my wife and I visited the !Kung San Bushmen in Botswana, Africa. The Kalahari Bush people are the stuff of legends, and we were thrilled to be able to spend several days learning from them. We lived as they currently live: as hunter gatherers. In human history, this is how we have lived for over 99% of our time on earth.

Our first morning with this group, we awoke to an early dawn in our tents and found that half of the Bushmen were already gone. Apparently a large bush buck had come through camp during the night and our new friends were in hot pursuit. On average, male Bushmen travel nine to ten miles per day, the women six to seven. Sometimes their hunt is successful, often times, as on our occasion, it wasn't. But the fact is that their movement capacity is vast, and it is all concerned with food.

Our Paleolithic ancestors lived in a fashion roughly similar to that of the contemporary Kalahari Bushmen. Hence our interest. It was during those millions of years when our great, great, great, great, etc. grandparents formed their biology—the gene sequences and signaling patterns which yield our present structure and function. Our present selves were shaped during these hundreds of thousands of generations of daily threat. To our forbearers, a constant imperative was "survive." And mobility was the key to that survival.

The Roots of Our Modern Diet

Our ape cousins lived predominantly on vegetable materials, leaves, roots and fruits. All of these have relatively low-calorie value per amount of mass ingested compared to meat, which is much more energy rich. But regardless of the amount of animal and plant proportions in the diet of our ancestor's, their food contained much more fiber content than most modern people's diets—another food issue of importance to diabetes.

It is also notable to conclude that the Bushmen (and hunter-gatherer ancestors) eat no purified carbohydrates other than honey, which they rarely happen upon by chance, and is highly prized. Similarly, the bony remnants of the prey animals on which Homo erectus feasted periodically revealed that Mr. and Mrs. Erectus particularly enjoyed the bone marrow because it was rich in fat content. Taste evolved to place unusual preference on these two types of food, honey and marrow fat, because they were the most highly-concentrated, caloric-dense portion of our ancestors' diet list. It is therefore understandable how our modern diets evolved.

Working for Your Dinner

Whatever was on the dinner table for Homo erectus got there, after much effort. It is estimated that our ancestors exerted 45% to 85% more energy than do current day people. A recent report in *Science* indicates that Neanderthals had huge appetites to feed their immense energy expenditures—5000 calories per day is their projected energy budget. Numerous authorities feel that the highly mobile nomadic persons were robust and healthy. They had to be. This evidence is provided by reference to the medical records of current aboriginal people. Primitive people who were not healthy are not our ancestors.

All of our ancestors were endurance athletes of the highest caliber. Their small communities and relative isolation shielded them from most infections. They died from not getting enough to eat or from being eaten by stronger and hungrier competitors.

Dental evidences reveal that Neanderthals, like present day Eskimos, commonly experienced periods of starvation when weight losses of 10% of body weight were common. Feast or famine was the pattern for most of mankind's prehistory.

The Transition to Modernity

So that was how things were for the great, great majority of mankind's time on this fertile planet. It was only 10,000 years ago that our ancestors abandoned their nomadic hunter-gatherer mode of life. They no longer hunted for food or were hunted as food. They grew it. For the first time, people had enough to eat, and things started to change in a hurry. The biggest change was a surge in population.

Jared Diamond's gemlike book, *Guns, Germs, and Steel* is a brilliant exposition of the mega forces unleashed by the constant food availability, first claimed in the Tigris and Euphrates Valley of Iraq and Iran. New social and governmental arrangements arose. Disease flourished because of the density of populations provided by caloric sufficiency. Exercise demands dramatically lessened, though being a farmer for most was still hard work. A leisure class now appeared—a designation unknown to the Bushmen.

Becoming Modern (and Fatter)

With global modernization and urbanization, dietary changes and a more sedentary lifestyle developed. As a result of a rise in car ownership, walking even short distances has decreased. In our homes, modern appliances, availability of ready-made foods, availability of television and computers have resulted in a decrease in manual labor, an increase in the use of high calorie convenience foods, and a decrease in the engagement in active recreational activities. Escalators and elevators have resulted in a decrease in the simple physical activity of climbing stairs. And as more and more of our open areas are populated, the accessibility of safe areas for walking and playing is diminishing. A British civil report indicated that between 1955 and 1990 there was a 65% decrease in personal energy expenditure, due to the adoption of many energy-saving devices and a more general use of the automobile.

After twenty years of acculturation, the muscle strength of Eskimos was found to be 35% decreased. Mechanized farming in Japan cut the work load by 50% and China recorded a 130% increase in cars in a 20-year period. Obesity rates have soared in China.

While attention was drawn to the dreadful famines which affected every continent of the earth, the truth is that the last several centuries have set the stage for worldwide obesity and thereby the global threat of diabetes.

Down Under

On another backpack expedition, this one to Australia, my wife and I stopped in for a courtesy visit to the district health officer in the outback oasis of Alice Springs. After initial pleasantries the local doctor, said "We're about to go broke." I was taken aback. He explained, "For 40,000 years, our native aborigines have been living bare-assed under the stars, pretty much cut off from the rest of us. We felt that this was just not right or dignified. So we invited and encouraged them to town. And drawn by the bright lights and financial incentives they meandered in, where they found McDonald's and the liquor store. And the rest is history. They gained many pounds, became totally sedentary, and developed diabetes, and as a result, progressively rotted their kidneys. So they are all now on kidney dialysis at $40,000 per person per year. We are going broke as a result."

Dr. Kerin O'Dea of the University of Melbourne tried a different strategy to combat the problem. She arranged for a small group of aborigines, who had already developed diabetes, to return home to the Outback. They resumed their Spartan diet, ate only food that they hunted or gathered. Kangaroo meat was the principal fare, and walked a lot. She re-contacted them several months later, and found that their weights had returned to normal and their diabetes had disappeared as clearly as did their future need for dialysis.

Worldwide Fat

Meanwhile in Africa and in the Middle East, the scenario is playing out in dramatic fashion. The December 29, 2004 *Wall Street Journal* featured a front-page article "New Obesity Boom in the Arab countries has Old Ancestry." It cited a table of the incidence of overweight and obesity in five Arab countries. In Bahrain, 83% of the women are overweight or obese.

Featured in the column was a story of a young woman in Mauritania, an impoverished nation in the Western Sahara. When she was eight, her mother began to force-feed her. On waking, she was forced to consume a gallon of milk, plus couscous. She had milk and porridge for lunch and later a full dinner. If she balked at eating her fare, her mother squeezed her toes. Now 38 years old and slim because of the family's inability to pay for the rich diet any longer, she maintains her belief in the practice of forced feeding of young women since "beauty is more important than health". Obesity is esteemed because it represents prosperity, beauty, and fertility.

This practice is called gavage, after the French practice of over-feeding geese to produce *foie gras*. Twenty-two percent of Mauritanian women were force-fed as young girls. Some grew so fat that they could barely move. The incidence of diabetes has soared.

The historical identification of obesity as a sexual attractant in this area has caught the attention of the World Health Organization, which is now instituting a broad series of counter-measures aimed at reversing the centuries' old cultural practices.

Finding Civilization ... and Getting Diabetes

The Pima Indians are of Mexican origin and are of supreme interest because they have developed the highest incidence of diabetes of any single group in the United States. Over 50% of them have diabetes. They didn't have any diabetes when they were running up and down mountainsides on the other side of the Rio Grande. Their trek north has done them in just like the Australian aborigines. Lack of physical activity and an increased intake of calories have resulted in obesity and diabetes. There must be a huge lesson in all of this somewhere, and the examples of this "displacement diabetes" are not confined to the Australian aborigines and Pimas. Jared Diamond wrote again about the little Pacific island of Naunu, which had zero diabetes until it "found" civilization. Westernization is dangerous to your health.

A crucial point to be made from the early historical evidence is that Type 2 diabetes was nonexistent or at least rare for thousands of years. Since our early years as humans, our genes have changed almost none at all. The fact that diabetes now sits astride our collective chests and beats on us suggests that this is not because of a mutation, but because of human-created circumstances. If we have created them, we should be able to un-create them, which is what this book is fundamentally about.

3

You Can Prevent Diabetes

It is far better not to crash your car than to crash it and have to deal with all the pain and indignity that is inflicted by the repair shop and insurance company, as they try to sort out whether the hostile truck, or tree, or you are to blame.

It is far better *not* to get diabetes in the first place than it is to tend it after it has started to flare.

"Doctor, I have a disease. Do something about it."

My reply could be: "What if what I have to help you isn't as good as what you can do for yourself." What if I give you a pain pill for the thumbtack in your foot when the best thing to do is for you to take the thumbtack out yourself?

Every book has a most important chapter that is most critical in establishing the goals and outcomes that the author hopes for in writing the book. For this book, this is that chapter. Whereas the surrounding chapters provide important background to many aspects of this raging crisis, it is this chapter that is central to the primary intent.

Mike McGinnis and Bill Foege's critical paper in the *Journal of the American Medical Association*, "Actual Causes of Death in the U.S.," makes the crucial point that the alleged big killers, heart disease, cancer, stroke, and diabetes are not actual causes of death. Instead, the real villains are underlying behavioral elements such as lack of physical activity, excessive calories, smoking and the like—which lead to these conditions. Looking at the "actual" causes of death, it becomes increasingly apparent that our only hope is prevention. That is where our attention must be focused.

With breathtaking speed, diabetes is increasing in incidence and severity. If uncontrolled, it will be irreversible and will surely exact a frightful toll of future human misery. Now knowing what we do about what causes diabetes, it is imperative strategy that we do all we can to keep it from spreading, and to limit its occurrence in the first place. This is prevention. This conclusion is not wishful thinking. Extensive international experimental studies show not only that diabetes can be prevented, but how to do it.

Pre-Diabetes

As indicated previously, we know that Type 2 diabetes' occurs only after a period of time during which a normal unsuspecting person silently harbors a sequence of subtle changes, that after a number of years leads to the diagnosis.

For 40 years, research workers have been probing relatives of diabetic persons with a variety of provocative tests to see whether there may be a precursor state which, if identified, could provide clues to the subsequent development of diabetes.

In 1967, two research workers at the famous Karolinska Institute in Stockholm, Rolf Luft and Erol Cerasi, coined the important term "pre-diabetes." They and their followers didn't actually know the details of what it represented, but the term indicated their intuition that there is an identifiable early stage in which real clues can be detected, and which portends later real trouble. The concept of pre-diabetes is analogous to other medical terms such as pre-cancer and pre-hypertension. What's hoped is that in identifying these three early stages of disease, actions may be taken to prevent the development of the disease before it is full-blown. This is what Pap smears are all about, and community screenings for unsuspected elevated blood pressure. The same reasoning applies to diabetes.

PRE-DIABETES DIAGNOSIS CRITERIA

Fasting blood sugar 100–125 mg/dl (5.6–6.9 mmol/l) Fasting—no food or drink for 8 hours or more.

A blood sugar of 140–199 mg/dl (7.8–11.1 mmol/l) two hours after drinking 75g glucose dissolved in water during a glucose tolerance test.

Since Luft and Cerasi's introduction of the term pre-diabetes in 1967, research workers have been trying to dissect the "early" steps in the development of Type 2. Such effort is clearly warranted. A 2004 estimate provided by Health and Human Services suggests that 41 million people within the age range of 40 to 74 are pre-diabetic. However, the total number is probably around 50 million.

Figure 7. **Progression to Type 2 Diabetes**

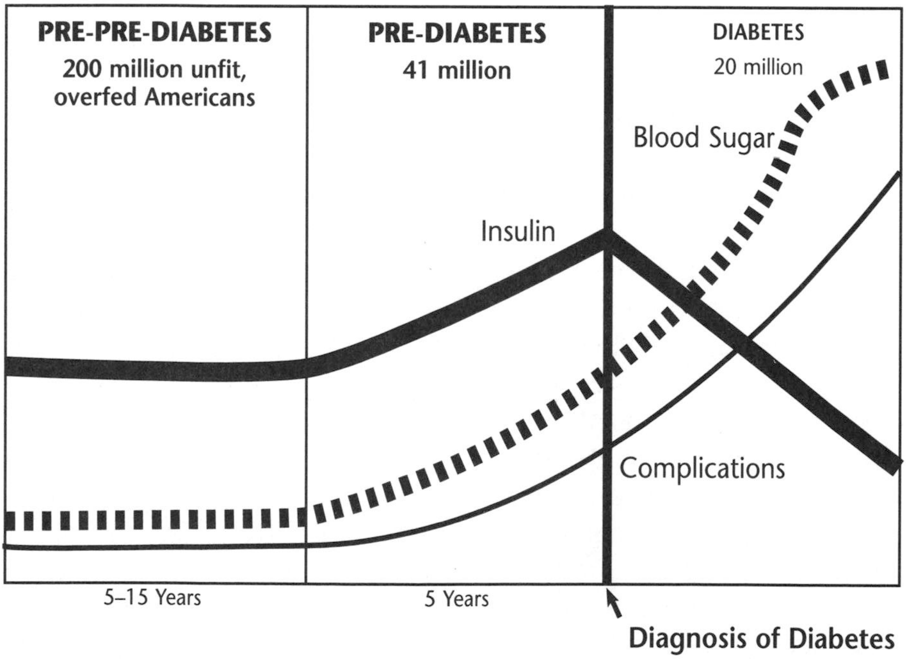

PRE-PRE-DIABETES	PRE-DIABETES	DIABETES
200 million unfit, overfed Americans	41 million	20 million

Blood Sugar

Insulin

Complications

5–15 Years   5 Years

Diagnosis of Diabetes

It is reasonable to suggest that there is an even earlier stage in the eventual discovery of Type 2. Before pre-diabetes comes pre-pre-diabetes, during which time the body is burdened with inactivity and overweight but is still able to keep the level of the blood sugar in the normal range. This sequence is displayed in Figure 7.

The Body's Struggle to Adapt

The research scientists at the Clinical Diabetes and Nutrition Section of the National Institutes of Health in Phoenix have been at the forefront of the effort to tease out the sequence of events that characterize pre-diabetes. Visiting there, I learned of their probing studies of the diabetic-susceptible Pima Indians. Their work employs a variety of techniques which allow measurement of most of the major contributors to carbohydrate and fat metabolism. They also have the capacity to measure the amount of physical activity that their experimental subjects are pursuing by means of a total body calorimeter—one of the few in the country. This hermetically-sealed study chamber allows the experimenters to trace every smidge that goes into and out of the body during the experimental period. Not only are the food and excretory products precisely measured, but the inspired and expired gases as well, so that an accurate balance sheet of the body's metabolism can be created.

Their methods provide measurements of how the fat, muscle tissue, liver, and beta cells are interacting. By observing the changes in their subjects over a period of months, they are able to decipher what comes first, what is cause and what is effect.

This group published a summary paper of their work in the *Journal of Clinical Investigation* in 1999. Four hundred and four members of the Gila River Indian community were enrolled in the study in 1998, with an average age of 26. At the onset of the study, a battery of tests was performed on them and the results reflected a normal metabolic pattern at that time. One hundred and fourteen of the group were evaluated and tested on at least three subsequent annual occasions. Thirty-eight of these individuals went on to develop Type 2 diabetes during a five-year observation. These 38 "progressors" were compared with 31 other "non-progressors," who did not develop diabetes during this interval. The interval between normal and pre-diabetes was 1.8 years, and 3.3 years from pre-diabetes to diabetes. So it took 5.1 years to get from normal to diabetes. A possible differentiating aspect was that the progressors gained twice as much weight as the non-progressors during the study. Weight gain was a powerful predictor of this sad sequence.

A logical story unfolds. Weight gain leads to increased fat deposits in the body fat stores, in the muscle cell, in the liver, and in the beta cells of the pancreas. This increased fat burden—the trailer full of cinder blocks—is evidenced by the increased traffic in fat as measured by the levels of free fatty acids (FFA) and triglycerides in the blood.

Higher blood fat levels decrease glucose utilization, which in turn leads to higher blood sugar levels. The pancreas' beta cells then need to pump out more insulin. As increased body fat provokes higher amounts of free fatty acids leading to decreased glucose, an elaborate new set of compensatory events begins. The human body struggles to adapt. Chemical mediators such as leptin, adiponectin, resistin, and a dozen other compounds are released by fat issues, the liver and blood cells. These are the elaborate micro-regulation occasioned by the switch from fat to carbohydrate and back again. The attempt to place all of these bodily reactions into a unified process occupies much current experimental effort in Arizona and throughout the world.

Not my Problem ... Or is it?

Inclusion of exercise in already complex experimental models makes a full investigational model of "real life" diabetes cumbersome and complicated. Because of this, exercise and its central participatory role in the whole process of diabetes is understudied.

We know that physical exercise has major effects on every step of the above proposed sequence and affects blood and glucose utilization and storage. It promotes insulin sensitivity and increases the sensitivity of muscle cell glucose transporters. Lack of exercise exaggerates the effects of obesity and insulin insufficiency. Therefore, the impaired glucose use of early diabetes is a double jeopardy situation comprised of too much fat and too little exercise. This is precisely the situation that is epidemic.

Obesity and physical inactivity leads to pre-diabetes, which leads to diabetes, which leads to destruction. One hundred and fifty million overweight and 200 million physically inactive leads to 41 million pre-diabetic and 20 million diabetics and how many pre-pre-diabetics?

Having developed a reasonable enough explanation for the blaze, the arson detectives write up a report containing their interpretations as to the origin of the fire.

This report was widely circulated, but initially it scarcely caused a ripple of public reaction. This reaction was either "This is someone else's problem, not mine," or "Even if it happens to me, my doctors will take care of it."

Don't believe it for a second, folks.

In Search of a Prevention Strategy

The Pima Indian report was heard loud and clear by Dr. David Nathan of Harvard, premier diabetes expert. He and over 400 scientists from 27 prestigious medical centers formed the Diabetes Prevention Program Research Group. They gathered all the supporting reports they could find concerning the "Why?" of the diabetes epidemic. Additionally, they asked, "What can we do about it, to minimize its spread, or possibly prevent it from happening at all?"

These experts decided on a dual strategy. To assess whether either or both could be found to respond to the "Why" question, they selected two approaches: a drug approach or a lifestyle approach, the latter utilizing exercise and diet.

In my view, the Diabetes Prevention Trial ranks among the most significant medical demonstrations of all time. It represents an important synthesis of public health and clinical medicine. It blends behavioral observations with pharmaceutical promise. Most of all, it reaches into the heart of the blaze that is raging and seeks a strategy that might divert the course of diabetes from its malevolent spread.

The trial's design was inspired. It addressed the assembly of scraps of information relevant to a prevention strategy. It did not seek for the reversal of firmly established damage, but asked instead whether by addressing an earlier phase of the disease the full flame might be averted.

The First Step for Those at Risk

From 1996 to 1999, the prevention study group recruited 3,234 participants, 70% with a family history of diabetes, average age 51, average weight 207, and average leisure time physical activity equal to 40 minutes of walking per week.

The subjects' selection was dependent upon their fasting blood sugar values, which were considered to be pre-diabetic.

This group was divided into three equal segments of 1,100 each. The first group received a placebo medication plus general advisories about diet and exercise with printed material and 20- to 30-minute individual sessions annually. The second group received the same lifestyle advisories plus metformin (glucophage). The third group, the intensive lifestyle intervention group, was intended to lose 7% of body weight, and was encouraged to do 150 minutes per week of moderate-intensity exercise, such as brisk walking. A 16- lesson curriculum was taught individually by case managers for the first 24 weeks and monthly thereafter. Group lessons with a case manager were utilized for further reinforcement of behavior change. Blood tests were obtained every six months with the primary intent of discerning who became diabetic and when. When a fasting blood sugar rose above 126 mg/dl, the diagnosis was changed from pre-diabetes to diabetes. The participants were followed an average of 2.8 years. After these years the control group weights were unchanged, the metformin group had on average lost four pounds. The life-style group had lost 12. After three years, the control and metformin groups' physical activity levels were unchanged. The life-style group, however, showed a 50% increase in physical activity.

This study was canceled in May 2001, a year earlier than originally targeted because of clear evidence of the effectiveness of the
two trial groups, the metformin and lifestyle cohorts compared to
the placebo group. The lifestyle group reduced the incidence of new
diabetes by 58%, the metformin group showed a 31% reduction as
seen in the accompanying graph.

Figure 8. **Incidence of Type 2 Diabetes During the Prevention Trial**

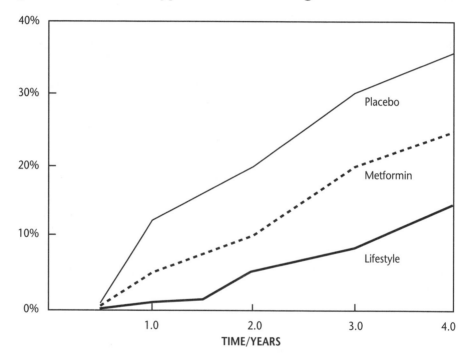

Along with the majority of informed readers of the data, I was
astonished. The actual amounts of weight lost and exercise increase
were modest but were sufficient within a brief period of 2.8 years
to reveal major benefits. To me, this report is one of the most significant papers in the world medical literature in the last 25 years.

The results were matched by similar studies from China, the Da
Qing study, and another from Finland. Three lifestyle diabetes
prevention reports represent a vigorous unambiguous answer to
the questions "What should we do?" and "How do we address
this epidemic?"

Reaction to this article was immediate and far-reaching. One of the most insightful was published in *Diabetes Care* by Thomas Buchanan of the University of Southern California School of Medicine. He made the important, qualifying point of asking whether the diabetes prevention trials cited above truly represented prevention. Might they instead only indicate a delay in the onset of the disease, a honeymoon? The relative short observation time of the trials was brief compared to the usual time of progression to the full-blown disease. He pointed out further that a portion of the metformin group displayed an accelerated incidence of diabetes after the drug was stopped, suggesting an effect on blood sugar without a corresponding effect on the progression to diabetes, which is the ultimate concern.

He concluded that "diet and exercise programs should be the first step in addressing high risk patients. Patients' whose glucose levels do not rise during a given behavioral intervention have achieved the goal of diabetes prevention, stability."

Amen.

Take Ownership

Critical for a diabetic's self-management success is taking ownership of the disease. Diabetes is with a person 24/7/365 and requires ongoing attention. If you have diabetes, your doctor, diabetes educator or health-care professional will provide the necessary tools to assist you in managing your own health care.

One plan does not fit all. You need not give up all the foods you like; instead, you must understand how to correctly incorporate these foods into your daily life. Knowledge is hugely important in diabetes management. That's why it's so very important for a diabetic to receive a referral for diabetes education.

Beyond the basics, diabetes education can also assist diabetics in their choice of glucometer—finding the one that best meets their specific needs. Maybe you want one with large numbers, while another person might want one with features tracking blood glucose levels, medication, insulin dose, and physical activity.

If you have diabetes, it is important that you take the tools provided—information about meal planning, glucose monitoring, and the importance of physical activity—and apply that knowledge to your daily life.

The Wrong Message

Being convinced of the great and overriding importance of prevention, I was distressed when I attended the International Congress on Diabetes meeting in Mexico City a few years ago. The meeting was held at the immense convention hall, directly across the street from the park. The entire frontage was festooned with huge banners proclaiming the competing virtues of a wide variety of diabetic medications. Inside, where the meetings took place and where the abstracts of research work were displayed, 95% of the lectures and papers concerned pharmacologic efforts to control diabetes. Almost no notice was given to preventive alternatives. A healthy lifestyle of diet and exercise is not where the money is. Sad but true.

4

Controlling Your Diabetes

When confronted by an epic tragedy of the scale of the recent Malaysia tsunami, it is logical to scan the doomsday headlines to search for some little story of safety within the ruin, hope amid the despair. We always look for the good news within the bad.

When considering if there is anything that is positive among the grim statistics and personal heartaches which accompany diabetes today, I am old enough and have seen enough of diabetes in my lifetime to give thanks for one aspect. And that is knowledge.

My first encounter with diabetes was when I was four or five years old, at the absolute most remote edge of my boyhood memory. I recall Granddaddy Welty, aged 62. I visited him with Mother, his daughter, in Greensburg, Pennsylvania, the ancestral home. He sat in the second-floor family room in an overstuffed armchair, his left leg up on a stool. The leg was gangrenous. It stank. When we visited, I wanted out of there.

Granddaddy refused to have his leg amputated. He died shortly thereafter. This is my only recollection of him. Not a happy memory, diabetes was etched into my little brain as a genuine piece of hell on earth.

That was 70 years ago. Treatment of diabetes then was extremely crude. Granddaddy suffered.

If Used, Knowledge Is Power

A general rule is that scientific knowledge doubles every ten years. My father used to delight in telling me of the dean's first lecture to the freshman at the Harvard Medical School. He said, "In the next four years, you will learn of the magnificent workings of the human body and what can go wrong with it. The problem, of course, is that ten years from now, half of what we teach you will no longer be true. And worse, we don't know which half that is."

If we had to confront the present diabetes epidemic armed only with the knowledge of my medical school days, the statistics would be even more staggering. We know much more today than then. That's the good news. But the figures shout the bad news. Obviously, other forces are dominating: the number of diabetics increases in spite of our great new knowledge.

We know a lot, but we don't know how to get people to change the way they have become accustomed to living. How do we raise awareness of the seriousness of diabetes?

If you get nothing else out of this book, I want you to realize that diabetes is deadly, but if you are in control, it doesn't have to be.

Knowledge is power, and you need to take control of this disease! I recognize that it is not easy, but as you read these pages, know that it will make a difference in the quality and quantity of your life.

Treatment Problems

The *hallelujah* moment of insulin discovery was dampened by a new problem. As a result of the zealous use of insulin, instead of high blood sugar there was now low blood sugar, hypoglycemia. This serious, sometimes fatal condition was caused not by the disease of diabetes, but by its treatment. It ushered in an entire new area of diabetes care.

Figure 9. **Blood Sugar and Insulin Levels**

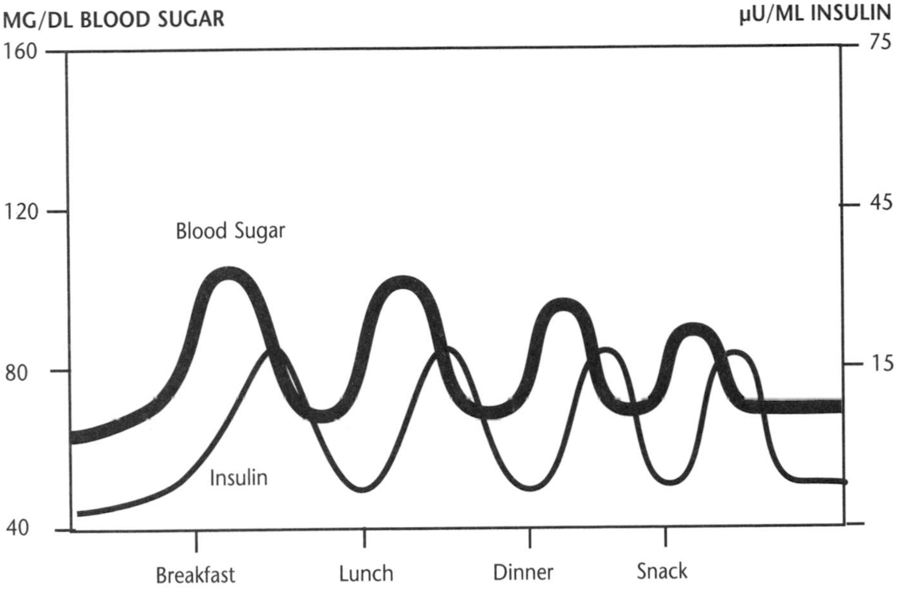

MG/DL BLOOD SUGAR   µU/ML INSULIN

For hundreds of years it had been known that in normal non-diabetic persons, blood sugar goes up-and-down according to the timing of the previous meal as shown in Figure 9.

With diabetes, the level of the blood sugar also varies, but at higher levels.

With the arrival of insulin a new consideration to the varying blood sugar levels was introduced.

Insulin provided a lid on the blood sugar going too high, but the new complication of too low, hypoglycemia, became yet another demon. Hypoglycemia is dangerous because diabetic persons are often unable to detect its early symptoms: weakness, sweating, and anxiety. Left untreated, hypoglycemia leads to unconsciousness as the brain is starved of its main fuel, glucose. Death can even occur. The treatment of hypoglycemia is simple. It is sugar, food.

Urine Testing

Back then the standard way of treating diabetes was to ask the patient to test her urine several times each day to see if it contained sugar. The test results were recorded in a diary which became the main discussion during a doctor's visit.

The presence of sugar in the urine was the measurement tool, because testing for the sugar level in the blood was confined to the doctor's laboratory. And even then, it proved of minor usefulness because of its variability. Assessing a month's worth of urine tests was valuable in guiding insulin dosage, although it was still a crude guess. Sugar spills over into the urine only when the blood sugar level is over 180 mg/dl.

So any sugar in the urine is bad; but no sugar in the urine, while ideal, also indicated that the level of blood sugar was below 180.

In the effort to keep the blood sugar in the normal range, certainly below 180, insulin was given. Unfortunately, there was no easy test for low blood sugar levels and insulin reactions became a serious issue. The term "brittle diabetes" was introduced to indicate those diabetics who had high blood sugar one moment and low the next. The low point became even more of a concern than the high because a person could still feel okay and function with high levels. But the margin for safety at the low end was slight and insulin reactions became problem number one.

I recall in my days as the camp doctor at Camp Firefly for diabetic children the ritual of waking the kids up in the middle of the night to be sure that their sugar levels were not too low.

With the terror of too low levels pervading, in the care of diabetes the dictum "spill a little" became the standard. It meant giving enough insulin to keep the lid on the high-level, but not enough to allow the bottom to drop out into insulin shock and hypoglycemia. Not too high, but certainly not too low was the mantra for 50 years.

High levels of blood sugar were tolerated because the reverse seemed worse. We became content with elevated levels of blood sugar.

This was the reality until 30 years ago. During these decades it became apparent that persons were no longer dying from diabetes directly. They were instead dying of terrible complications associated with it. However, the connections between diabetes and its complications were not clear, or at least not conclusive.

Self-Monitoring Blood Sugar

In the last 20 years a powerful new tool has emerged, one vastly superior to the urine monitoring strategy. This is self-monitoring of the blood sugar levels. This simple, reliable technique has proven to be revolutionary in the management of diabetes.

No longer is the patient flying blind. At the ready is an immediate answer as to the level of the blood sugar. This assessment tool is universally accepted as the standard of management. Several companies compete for the label of "best" blood glucose monitor. Most significantly is the availability and use of the test.

No single rule applies for the recommended frequency of testing, but, in general, more is preferable to less. Anyone using insulin should be more attentive, but anyone who is changing any aspect of their care package should check several times each day. The knowledge provided by this technology is invaluable. Continuous glucose monitoring has also been instrumental in determining blood glucose trends over the course of days. Efforts are underway to combine a continuous monitoring system with an insulin pump to further advance blood sugar control with a minimum of low blood sugar reactions.

Using Knowledge and Data to Take Control

Blood glucose monitoring is essential for individuals with diabetes. However, it must be used as a tool for improved control, not just a depository for numbers. Monitoring provides accurate information about your blood sugar at a specific point in time; it reflects your food choices, your physical activity, and the effectiveness of your medication and or insulin regimen. A diabetic should look at their numbers as information for them to help manage their disease.

Look for patterns which will assist you in better management. For example, if blood glucose levels are always high before lunch, you may want to engage in some form of physical activity in the morning to lower them.

Or you may want to evaluate *what* you eat for breakfast. Are you drinking juice or eating a piece of fruit? Due to its fiber content, a piece of fruit will not elevate your blood glucose levels as high as the glass of juice. Perhaps you opt for half a bagel rather than the whole thing. Or perhaps you could observe the effect of a high-fiber cereal rather than a sugared cereal. Choosing the former will improve your control and assist with weight loss.

Another effective means of gaining understanding (as well as control) of your diabetes is to investigate the many relevant computer programs available. They can help track your blood glucose levels, your nutrition and exercise programs, as well as your medications and activities.

You could keep a log detailing all the important facts (blood sugar levels, nutrition, exercise, medication, and stress). This is a very effective way to gain both understanding and control of diabetes.

Hemoglobin A1C

Thirty years ago, research workers at Harvard discovered that the common hemoglobin molecule found in the red blood cells had an affinity for glucose. Their binding produced a compound labeled "glycosylated hemoglobin"—or "Hemoglobin A1C" for short. The advantage of this new measurement tool was that its value reflected a composite value of all the blood sugars of the preceding three months. Hemoglobin A1C quickly became the gold standard for patient and physician alike for use as blood sugar control. It provided a reliable tool to understand what was really going on, not just at a moment but over an extensive period of time. See Figure 10 to determine the A1C level and corresponding blood sugar levels.

This binding of blood sugar to hemoglobin is only a single example of sugar linking to many different protein molecules, called glycoproteins. When the blood sugar level is normal, the amount of these glycoproteins that are produced is small. However, when sugar levels rise in uncontrolled diabetes, they rise to abnormal amounts. Since glycoproteins circulate through the blood, when their levels rise they accumulate in the tiniest blood vessels, the arterioles and capillaries—much

Figure 10. **Reaching Target**

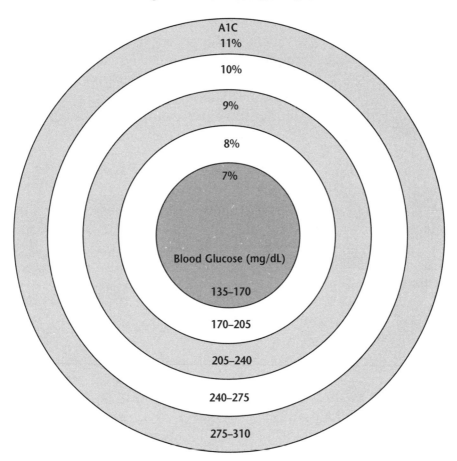

A1C
11%

10%

9%

8%

7%

Blood Glucose (mg/dL)

135–170

170–205

205–240

240–275

275–310

Normal Hemoglobin A1C is < 6% (135 mg/dL)
American Diabetes Association recommends < 7% (170mg/dL)
American College of Endocrinologists recommends ≤ 6.5% (152mg/dL)

like sludge in a small stream. This gunk then blocks normal circulation and leads to widespread vascular occlusion. The blood supply gets "gummed up," which can actually be seen through an ophthalmoscope. Similarly, the blood vessels to the kidney, the brain, to the entire body are plugged by this abnormal material.

Getting the Maximum Benefit from Your Medications

The United Kingdom's Prospective Diabetes Study dramatically proved that the management of blood sugar, A1C levels, blood pressure and cholesterol are all intertwined. For the diabetic to reduce the risks of complications, it is important that all of these factors are under control. Simultaneously addressing this variety of conditions can get burdensome and complicated. Medication regimens to correct abnormalities may be complex and expensive. However, it is absolutely critical that individuals with diabetes work closely with their physician to find a medication regimen that can be consistently maintained.

It's not uncommon for a patient with diabetes to be taking three different oral medications: blood pressure medication, cholesterol-lowering medication and diabetes medications. It is important that you take these prescribed medications consistently: they are important in the control of blood sugar, blood pressure and cholesterol.

If you have difficulty remembering to take medication, develop a reminder system. Use a pill box, keep a calendar, or post a note in a significant location that will assist you in establishing a routine.

Timing of medications may also be important. So discuss with your doctor and pharmacist any special requirement or directions. For example, glipizide should be taken on an empty stomach 30 minutes before the meal. And you cannot chew any sustained-release tablets, they must be swallowed.

Knowing how to correctly take your medication will help you gain their maximum benefit.

Important Studies

Accordingly, several large, highly controlled, excellent studies were performed in the United States, Sweden, Britain, and Japan. In 1993, the *New England Journal of Medicine* published the results of the American and Swedish studies. Both involved patients with Type 1 diabetes. The American experiment was begun in 1983 and involved 29 medical centers around the U.S. One thousand four hundred and forty-one Type 1 patients were followed for an average of 6.5 years. Part of the group had no detectable complications of any sort. Another group had mild eye and kidney change. Half the group was termed "the intensive therapy group," the other group was "the conventional therapy group." The conventional therapy group received one daily dose of insulin plus regular diet and exercise advice. They were examined every three months.

In contrast, the intensive therapy group received insulin three or four times each day by injection or external pump. The insulin doses were adjusted regularly according to four-time daily blood glucose monitoring results. The goal of therapy for this group was to reduce the fasting sugar levels to the 70 to 120 mg/dl range, and hemoglobin A1C to 6.5. The intensive group patients were seen at least once per month.

Ninety-five percent of the patients completed the study. Ninety-five percent of the scheduled appointments were kept. The mean of all blood sugar levels of patients in the intensive group was 155 as compared with 231 for the conventional group. Even more important were the results of the A1C, the levels of which were 8.8 for both groups at the start. The intensive group lowered their A1C to 6.9 whereas the conventional group rose slightly to 9.1.

The improvement in levels of sugar and A1C resulted in the desired improvements in rates of eye, kidney, and nerve complications, and in some cases, they were eliminated. These patients continue to be studied in order to assess the long-term benefit of intensive therapy. Follow-up has shown that those in the intensive treatment arm continue to demonstrate a lower incidence of complications.

The smaller Swedish study, with 102 patients, followed a similar protocol with conventional and intensive insulin schedules. Eight year follow-up results were reported. The A1C results of the intensive group was 9.5 originally and 7.1 at the conclusion. The conventional group results were 9.4 to 8.5 at the conclusion. Similar reductions in complications were reported.

Both studies reported that significant low blood sugar reactions were two to three times more common in the intensively treated group than in the conventional treatment group. But there was less than one case per patient year. Nonetheless, this feature caused concern about extending the implications of intensive therapy even further.

A further downside of the intensively treated group was the fact that these subjects gained considerably more weight, ten pounds, than the conventional group. The impact of this fact on longer term results remains to be seen.

Studies were done by the British and Japanese to determine if similar interventions would benefit Type 2 diabetics. Since 50% of newly diagnosed Type 2 patients already have evidence of complications at the time of their diagnosis, this issue was particularly pressing. This is why the Diabetes Prevention Trial was so critical.

The U.K. Prospective Diabetes Study Group enlisted 5,102 patients with Type 2 diabetes. Again, an intensive therapy regimen was used in half, incorporating a variety of treatments designed to lower sugar levels to a normal range. The conventional crew was managed largely with diet, with drugs used only if complications ensued. The average age of the group was 53.

Like the results of the American and Swedish Type 1 trials, both the fasting blood sugar values and the A1C levels were reduced by the intensive protocols. The intense protocols also provoked more low blood sugar values and weight gain similar to the Type 1 studies. It was found that not only was it critical to control blood sugar, but also lowering cholesterol and blood pressure was important in reducing complications. The intense treatment group resulted in a 25% reduction in eye, kidney, and nerve complications.

The smaller Japanese Type 2 trial used two insulin schedules and a 15-year observation period. Once again, marked improvement was found in the intensive treatment group.

Whereas the above four studies assessed the development of new small vessel disease and the associated complications, there is other evidence that even if such eye, kidney, and nerve disease is already established, stringent efforts at sugar control may delay or prevent further deterioration.

Figure 11. **Type 2 Diabetes and Heart Disease Deaths**

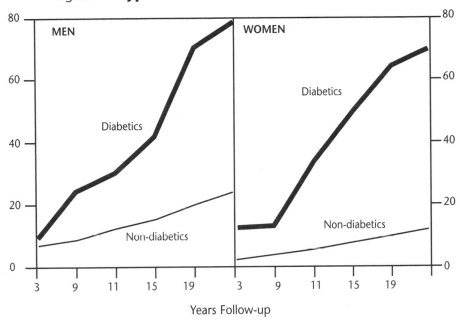

Years Follow-up

Heart Disease Risk

As noted in the graph above, 75% of persons with diabetes die from some cardiovascular complication.

Our arteries are like a tree, the trunk is the aorta, the big artery that emerges from the left, pumping, ventricle of the heart. The trunk splits progressively into smaller arteries which provide blood to every corner of the body. These large and medium arteries are prone to the development of atherosclerosis in which the tubes become clogged with chunks of cholesterol, inflammatory material, and clot. This is "large vessel disease," to which everyone is prone as seen in Figure 12.

The diabetic, however confronts not only large vessel disease, but the clogging of the smaller branches and twigs, the arterioles and capillaries, by the glycoprotein gum noted above.

This blockage brings its own set of problems, so that the diabetic is at double jeopardy of large and small vessel disease.

Persons with diabetes have double the risk of macrovascular (big vessel) death than non-diabetics. A person with diabetes

Figure 12. **Large Vessel Disease**

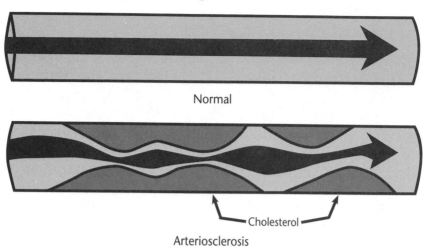

Normal

Cholesterol

Arteriosclerosis

experiencing the typical degree of atherosclerotic seen with diabetes, is at greater risk because of the added burden of small vessel disease. Two papers appeared in the *Annals of Internal Medicine* in 2004 that address this issue, one from Johns Hopkins and another from Great Britain. The Hopkins paper consisted of a survey of 13 studies of Types 1 and 2 diabetes, correlating hemoglobin A1C levels with cardiovascular death events, heart attacks and stroke. The authors concluded that higher A1C levels did predict a 15% to 20% increased risk of large vessel disease complications in persons with diabetes.

The British study went further. In their survey of 10,000 persons followed for eight years, there were 521 deaths and 806 vascular "events." They found a 1 point increase in A1C levels increased the risk of death by 25%. Further, this connection was present even in persons without diabetes. Or at least their glucose levels did not reach the criteria of definite diabetes, questionably pre-diabetes. Both articles indicate that there is more to atherosclerotic large vessel disease than cholesterol levels, high blood pressure, smoking, and the other traditionally cited risk factors. It seems clear to me that the common risk factor of physical inactivity could be responsible for a large part of this shared predisposition.

The Importance of Control

The diabetic control story has come full circle. When insulin was introduced in 1922, great relief was afforded to the very high sugar levels previously encountered. This was the first post-insulin era. However, because of the common occurrence of insulin reactions the medical profession backed off from their initial enthusiasm for normalization of the blood sugar levels. "Spill a little" sugar became the motto of the second era. This era also eventually passed because of the absolute proof that even modest abnormalities of blood sugar levels can increase the incidence of the dreaded combination of small vessel disease and the higher incidence of large vessel disease, including heart attacks and stroke. Therefore, we have come full circle back to the standard of tight control.

Tight control is not an easy job. Among other things, it requires skill, determination, knowledge, courage, optimism, persistence, patience, humor, and support from family and friends. While not easy, it has been made easier with the simple monitoring systems now available for frequent personal measurement of blood sugar levels. This is a huge advance.

New Therapies

The other big advance has been in the new insulin and drugs which have arrived recently on the scene. With judicious combination of insulin and oral agents, the dreaded complications of hypoglycemia can be managed and better sugar control approached. Low blood sugars can be minimized (but probably not totally avoided), since tight control inevitably means walking a fine line.

Each of these steps is now characterized in great detail, and each has become a potential step for further treatment. Some medications affect the absorption of glucose in the gut. Others direct their action to the peripheral burning of sugar in the tissues. Some affect sugar release by the liver and others make insulin more reactive at the tissue level. Finally, some medications work directly on the beta cells of the pancreas, making them more efficient in their insulin-producing action. What emerges is a total land, sea, and air attack on diabetes—with different agents working on different targets.

Ever since insulin was discovered, efforts have been made to increase the therapeutic options. Different types of insulin permitted a much more tailored approach to periods of greater need. More recently, further molecular modification of insulin itself allows an even greater range of options, a progress which shows no signs of letting up.

With the sulfonylurea drugs in the 1950s and 60s, clinicians used the opportunity for combining drugs with insulin. These drugs quickly grew into a whole array of drugs with different times of action. Then came a series of other medications, each designed to attack a particular step of glucose metabolism. The latest in the armature of medications are a new class of drugs which mimics the hormones released in response to food in the regulation of glucose. Amylin works to reduce the production of glucagon and is used to control blood sugar levels at meal time.

Combination Therapy

The rapidly enlarging range of options creates problems as well as opportunities. There are already articles appearing in the medical literature complaining of the mixing of apples and oranges in different proposed treatment schedules. It becomes increasingly difficult to compare one set of treatments with another unless much care is taken to insure the comparability of the different protocols.

A recent issue of *Diabetes Care* presented a series of articles concerning triple therapy. Current medical literature teems with early reports of other anti-diabetes drug combinations.

Regardless of which single program is selected, it should represent what is called "treating to target," which really means getting the hemoglobin AIC level to 6.5. Of course, one of the downsides of combining treatments is cost. Another is side effects. The more medicines one takes, the greater risk of side effects, either from the pill itself or from an interaction with other medications. Taking three or more different medicines makes it difficult to keep track of mischief.

Further, we know that people aren't very reliable in how they take pills. If they're not good at taking one kind, how would they be taking two or three? The more complicated things become, the more errors there are. It is therefore critical that individuals are well-educated as to the action and duration of their medications so that they are taken correctly and at the proper time. Unfortunately, many individuals with diabetes have no understanding of how their medications work and, as a result, may be taking them at the wrong time, or at a time when they may not achieve the optimal results. It is important to have an in-depth understanding of what any medication does, and how it will impact blood sugar. Prescriptions should also be filled in a timely fashion.

And never forget that exercise and healthy eating, important life-long changes, are crucial in an effective treatment. No matter what program is selected, the aim should be an A1C of 6.5 or lower. Beyond 6.5 is diabetes danger.

Control is back as a gold standard, but prevention is still the first major goal. If prevention fails, the fallback position is making the best of a tough situation.

One of my closest friends is 64 years old. He has had Type 1 diabetes for 35 years. By every criterion, he has no evidence of complications of any sort. He lives an extremely physically active life and is absolutely meticulous about his monitoring and insulin adjustment. He flirts with hypoglycemia constantly. We collectively celebrate how he has "beaten" diabetes.

But his case is the rarity. It is indisputably true that we know that control of sugar levels is crucial and we know how to do this. This failure to exploit our knowledge is unquestionably the cause of the dreadful 15 years shorter lifetime of diabetics compared to the average. Despite the increase in knowledge and treatment of diabetes, knowledge alone is insufficient.

Losing Control

First, we know that children with Type 1 tend to run a one plus higher average level of hemoglobin A1C because of the aforementioned fear of low blood sugar reactions. Second, though it is known that A1C levels should be below 7, where the risk of complication decreases, the number of persons reaching this goal is extremely low.

Maintaining A1C levels at a range of 6.5 - 7.0 is a tough order, particularly in light of the widespread evidence of very poor control of sugar levels elsewhere. A large Finnish survey provided additional information as to the low levels of blood sugar control in diabetic patients. Three thousand one hundred and ninety-five diabetic patients and 76 clinics were surveyed. The mean A1C level was 8.6, only 25% were under 7.3. Ten percent were over 11.2. Less than 10% of the A1C levels in this group were normal. The BMI levels correlated highly with A1C levels—once again linking obesity and diabetes.

The totally unacceptable levels were shocking. Bad news also exists in the United States regarding control. Dr. Lawrence Blonde of the American Association of Clinical Endocrinologists released statistics from 2003–2004, at the 2005 annual meeting. These results were discouraging. Two-thirds of all diabetics do not have their blood sugar under control. Even worse, these patients are unaware they are not in control. A recent Harvard University and University of North Carolina generated study reported management patterns of Types 1 and 2 diabetes in 30 American academic medical centers where medical care should approach the highest standards. One thousand seven hundred and sixty-five patient records were reviewed. The results were dismal. Whereas testing for important measures was excellent, there was a terrible response to the high level of poor test results. Only 34% of the patients met A1C level guidelines, only 10% of 1,765 surveyed patients met three basic clinical goals similar to the lack of improvement in hemoglobin A1C levels between 1988 and 2000. Worse was that only 40% of those with abnormal tests resulted in any adjustment of the control efforts.

Of greater concern is the lack of treatment change by health care providers to improve control. This laxity has been labeled "clinical inertia," and is being increasingly surveyed.

In 2001, the Diabetes Quality Improvement Project was initiated to seek ways of addressing this inertia. The results of the 1999 to 2000 National Health and Nutrition Examination Survey

(NHANES) showed no improvement in the last 12 years. A double problem is identified. Not only are A1C levels markedly and widely abnormal, little effort is being directed to their improvement. The United States, Finland, and the rest of the world have a long way to go to improving control.

Control is poor and effort to improve it is even worse. Knowing what to do is not the issue. Dealing with it is. So what's the problem?

Awarding a Well-Fought Battle

In contrast to these grim statistics is the presence of the Joslin Diabetes Victory Award System. The justifiably renowned Joslin Clinic in Boston proudly presents 25, 50, and 75 year awards to the Type 1 persons who have lived that long with no complications.

A September 22, 2004 press release told of medal awards to Robert and Gerald Cleveland, brothers from Jamesville, New York. They have lived for 78 and 72 years respectively, with Type 1 diabetes. In presenting the awards, Dr. George King, Director of Research at Joslin, said "To put their accomplishments into perspective, the Cleveland brothers developed diabetes shortly after the discovery of insulin and more than 70 years later, neither has developed any serious complications. Both are to be commended for meticulously managing their blood glucose levels. Day in and day out. For decades. They serve as an inspiration for anyone living with Type 1 diabetes." Bravo, Robert and Gerald!

Since the origin of the awards in 1970, 2,200 people have been celebrated for 50 years of diabetes control. Robert and Gerald are the 15th and 16th to be granted 75 year awards.

A similar award exists in Great Britain which is called the "Golden Years Cohort" for Type 1 patients who have had their disease for 50 years. There are now 400 awardees. Their average age at diagnosis was 14 years. Their current average age is 69. Winners tend to be lean and have low cholesterol values. Their A1C levels average 7.6. This recognition increases the sense of responsibility when we see that this serious disease with its serious complications and outcomes can be dealt with. Grim outcomes may be less Fate than Choice.

I Think I Can, I Know I Can ... I Do!

We at Stanford are fortunate to have as one of our stellar col-leagues, Professor Albert Bandura. His works are the most cited in the psychology literature. He is often included in lists of the most influential scientists of the past century. Albert's field is self-effi-cacy, the study of personal control and competency. He investi-gated the world of phobias (fear of snakes, flying, etc.), and from this he has written *the* book on behavior change. His work shows repeatedly that merely *knowing* what should be done is insuffi-cient. Building the belief in what should and can be done is where the action is.

The opposite of a well established sense of self-efficacy is the helpless-hopeless syndrome studied by Martin Seligman. Too often the person with diabetes adopts the forlorn and forbidding attitude of "It's beyond me." This is lethal. Judith Rodin, past president of the University of Pennsylvania and a highly regard-ed psychologist wrote, "Control is more likely to affect health than health is to affect control." The first step in sugar control is self control. "I think I can, I know I can, I do." This sequence can-not be put in a capsule, or a prescription written, or within a syringe. But it can be taught.

Bandura writes a prescription for self-efficacy much as I write a prescription for penicillin. His Rx has 4 parts. See Figure 13.

I learned this prescription 15 years ago, and regularly employed it whenever a patient has said to me, "I can't do that." Bill Henry, a 63-year-old gas station operator came to me as a patient several years ago because of fatigue. At 5 foot 9 inches, he weighed 216 pounds. His blood pressure was on the edge. A sometime smoker, television was his favorite exercise. His blood sugar value came back as 293. He was diabetic.

I brought Bill and his thirty-eight-year old wife in for the fol-low-up visit the next week, and revealed his diagnosis. This mat-tered a lot for Bill, but even more for his wife and two-year-old son. It was an emotional visit as Bill stared his uncertain future in the face. He silently set out with a new resolve.

He vanished from my practice for over a year, but reappeared a new person. His weight was 170, he looked fit, he had stopped smoking altogether, had joined some buddies at the YMCA for regular handball workouts. His blood sugar was normal.

He had followed Bandura's prescription of small steps of mastery, (a little at a time), peer examples (the Y), and social persuasion (he was knowledgeable about diabetes and its dangers). He had worked through his tough spots (cues of failure). Bill would

Figure 13.

Walter M. Bortz II, MD

Ph.: **333-333-3333**

Name: **200 Million Americans At Risk**

Date: **11/1/05**

R̽   PRESCRIPTION FOR SELF-EFFICACY

1. Small steps of mastery.

2. Peer examples.

3. Social persuasion and education,

4. The diminishment of cues of failure.

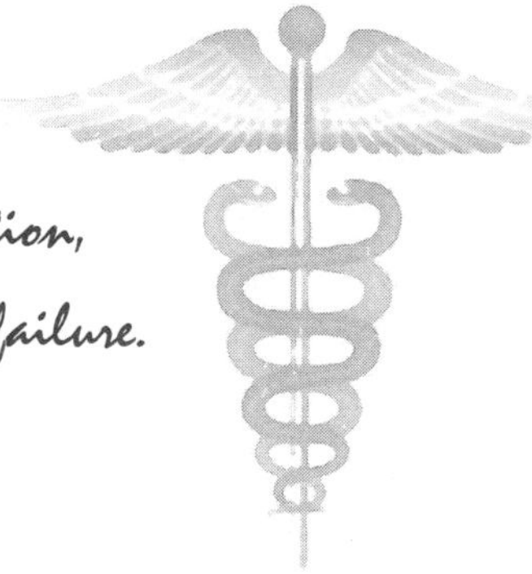

Refill **Many** times

Walter M. Bortz MD

Signature

live to see his son grow to manhood, not because of me, but because he had taken a full dose of "self-efficacy."

Several studies published on these themes have shown that the level of self-efficacy as determined by a battery of psychological profile tests correlates better with A1C levels than does knowledge. This affirms the statement that knowledge by itself is less important than taking control, owning your own health behavior. Not only is it important to provide information to patients, but additional strategies must be used to motivate and assist them in dealing with this disease. Intelligence and knowledge are lesser predictors of diabetes control than actually applying that knowledge in day to day living. Who is in control—diabetes or *you?*

Crisis Management

Stress is a major factor in the establishment of personal self-efficacy. The highly-stressed, unsupported person has much less of a chance of maintaining control, and becomes a sitting duck for diabetic complications. Dr. Richard Rubin of Johns Hopkins University is a master of illustrating the adverse effects of a stressed lifestyle on diabetic complications.

It is easy to say "Don't worry about that, only sweat the big things," but implementing that strategy in this fast-paced world is tough. With dozens of diabetic patients, I have established an excellent control situation only to have a life-stress intervene, and all measurements go crazy.

One of my patients lost his job. His son was a senior in high school and wanted to go to college. This guy had successfully managed his diabetes for seven years without a problem, but suddenly his blood sugar levels were through the roof. After several counseling sessions and medication adjustments, his levels began to stabilize. On his last visit, he had found two jobs, his son was graduating, his plans for college were in place, and his stressors were gone. He was now experiencing hypoglycemia and his medications were once again readjusted—downward this time. Crises must be managed not just by medical interventions, but by a renewed effort to extend and sustain self-efficacy.

Bandura has been an advocate of the use of technology to build self-efficacy. One of his pet projects in this regard for diabetics involves a Nintendo game, *Packy and Marlon,* designed "to improve a young person's self-confidence and ability and motivation to understand the rigors of care necessary to control insulin dependent diabetes."

In a control study of the effect of this video game on young persons with diabetes, its use decreased unscheduled urgent visits to the physicians by 75%. It also improved parental communication and increased self-efficacy with regard to diabetes. In the game, players win points by responding to challenges to the super-hero's diabetic health by hostile forces.

It's true that an ounce of prevention is worth many tons of cure. However, if the diabetic demon still escapes your efforts designed to shoo him away you should understand that tight control is the only acceptable control strategy. Such control derives from multiple sources.

"I have a disease. Doctor, do something for me."

What if your disease is best managed by a vigorous physical activity program and an enlightened eating pattern? I can't do that for you. Only you can own these behaviors. I can't prescribe them."

And what if you accept the responsibility and despite your best efforts, it doesn't work? Then and only then should the doctor get out the prescription pad. A prescription should be the last resort, not the first resource. In my professor of medicine's first lecture, he said, "I have done a lot more good by stopping medicine than by starting it."

Beyond Prescriptions

Even if medicines are started, the goal should be to reduce their strengths and their use altogether if possible. My personal gold standard for the medical care of diabetes patients is to prevent and limit the complications with as little or no medical intervention as possible.

As your fireman, what do I have to quench your diabetes fire? Such tools are of two predominant types, low-tech and high tech: pills and shots. The shots, of course, are insulin, the single most important compound in the entire world of diabetes control. Insulin rules. We must together protect it, insure it, encourage it and provide it via shots, if necessary.

Pills are insulin helpmates. Diabetes pills, in all shapes and descriptions, are each differently designed to support insulin's benevolent action. Some of these help the islet cells of the pancreas make more insulin. Some work to reduce the mechanisms which cause insulin resistance. Some help insulin to become more effective on the muscles, liver, and brain. Some work to decrease appetite or the chemical messengers which affect appetite. Some work to block food absorption.

Balancing Risk and Benefit

The pharmaceutical companies are eagerly on the lookout for improvement of the pills and for new pills to make insulin's action more effective. But even with improvements, the truth remains that all of these have side effects.

So use of pills must balance risk and benefit.

It is the high-tech capacities of the fire department that make the headlines. These approaches are at the leading edge of high science and are directed mostly to those with Type 1 diabetes. You might ask if insulin is so central to diabetes, why not just transplant its source into the body, to replace the defective part? That is what a good auto mechanic would do. Fair enough suggestion, but it is not that simple. Surgical transplant of a new pancreas, often from a motorcycle crash victim, is now a well-validated procedure performed it many medical centers, perhaps 1,000 per year nationally. Its usefulness as a major answer to the Inferno is limited, however, largely by the lack of availability of donor pancreases, despite intensive publicity recruitment strategies.

Aligned with the pancreas transplant technology is another high-tech strategy: islet cell transplants. This approach, while surgically less demanding still suffers from the problem of lack of donor tissue—even more so, since many of the islets are lost during the transfer handling. Research also exists to develop a long-term, drug-free protocol using pig islet xenotransplants as an alternative to human islet cell transplants.

Both whole pancreas and islet cell transplant tools require post-operative treatment with potent drugs, which bring an abundance of major complications with them. Recognizing this, some centers, including NIH, have abandoned islet cell efforts. Instead, they are focusing on the new frontier of stem cells, which hopefully can be harvested from the intended recipient thereby avoiding the risk of the drugs involved in preventing transplant rejection phenomena. It's hoped that these stem cells can be encouraged to take on a beta cell function. This area of science is only in its infancy and will unquestionably generate its own special kinds of problems. Wait and see.

And then there's the matter of money. These high-tech approaches are expensive, usually over $100,000 per person for the first year alone. With the surging incidence of diabetes, these costs become increasingly important. For most of the globe, which is similarly sharing the diabetes inferno, even the costs of insulin and pills are more than many people can afford.

Who's in Charge?

The Fire Department, with all its tools, is a secondary and insufficient player. Even at their best, all the diabetes pills, shots and transplants will not take care of everything. There is simply no avoiding the conclusion that a diabetic's total participation in their treatment is the central issue.

You need to take control.

5

Supersized Me

The next chapter is about energy out, in the form of movement. This chapter is the other side of the equation: energy in, food. In nature, movement and food are inextricably linked. However, one key difference between the two is how we view them: We hate to move, but we love to eat. This imbalance of our primitive inclinations creates the diabetic tumult which currently threatens our globe.

Think of it this way. Assuming the general average intake is 2,000 calories of food per day, times 365 days per year, an average individual eats 730,000 calories per year. In order for weight to stay stable we must move an equivalent amount or our weight will change. If we move more than we eat, we lose weight. If we move less than we eat, we gain weight.

Professor Jim Hill tells us that on average we gain 2 pounds of fat each year. One pound of fat is equivalent to 3,500 calories; therefore instead of eating 730,000 calories we actually eat 737,000 calories, which is 20 extra calories per day. Or, alternatively, we move 7,000 calories or 240,000 steps less per year or 660 steps less per day. Any combination of more food and less movement equals 2 pounds per year. But the point is that the energy-in energy-out balance is extraordinarily finely tuned. Twenty more calories in per day or 660 steps less per day, over the year, becomes the 2 pounds of weight gain.

A Modern Imbalance

The human body is a wonder of balance. The traditional word for this balance is homeostasis, a helpful term coined a hundred years ago by my dad's Harvard Medical School professor, Walter Cannon. Personally, I prefer the new term homeo-dynamics proposed by my good friend, Gene Yates, at the UCLA School of Medicine. Homeo-dynamics captures the world of competing and complementing chemical reactions which occur by the billions per second in the cells of our bodies.

How the whole affair is so magnificently tuned is as much cause for wonder as anything in the universe. For thousands of years, the balance of energy for humans was on the deficit side: too few calories in for the calories spent. Times have changed, and we are witnessing an imbalance of a different sort.

Figure 14. **Weight Balance**

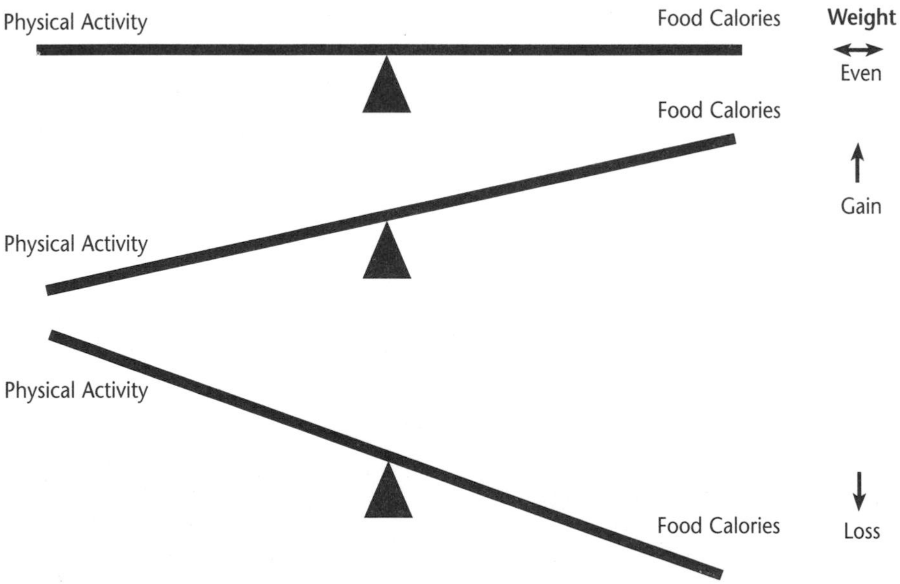

Diabetes Is *Not* Our Biological Destiny

Obesity is a new event. Diabetes is a new event. These observations actually offer reasons to be optimistic. If nature had ordained that our destiny was to be fat and diabetic, we would have a hard time finding a solution. But since these phenomena are so new it means that the diabetes inferno is not a natural act, and we therefore should be able to extinguish it by a concerted effort.

The energetic imbalance that we now encounter has two aspects: in and out. What has happened in only the last few decades to our caloric intake? Some experts claim our food consumption is no different than it was a hundred years ago, and so therefore, the epidemic is entirely inactivity driven.

Most experts agree however, that the intake side of the balance is also a significant contributor.

A February 2004 report from CDC indicated that between 1971-2000 women increased their daily caloric intake by 22%, men by 7%, (from 1,542-1,877 calories for the women, and from 2,450-2,618 calories for the men).

We have become zoo animals. We were born free on the Serengeti, but we now live the lives of caged animals. Our keepers come by periodically and throw some food at us. They know that domesticated animals must be very carefully fed. What once was an automatic regulation has been distorted by our enforced inactivity.

Chimps in captivity remain active and do not become obese, but our orangutan and gorilla cousins become lethargic, morose, and fat. When a wild animal stops moving, it usually risks starvation. But in our case, we are in danger of obesity. With such a nutritional calamity at hand, we should be fortunate to have experts in addressing the threat.

And we got 'em, billions of experts. Virtually everybody considers herself a food expert. Everyone has a theory largely based on personal preferences, filled with rationalizations.

When the average person seeks the right diet, he is confounded by the sheer number of supposed experts. How many different food pyramids have we had in the last 20 years? Contradictions abound which inevitably result in loud commercial claims for "The Diet to End All Diets."

Weight-loss books top the bestseller lists, each promising salvation between the book covers. With so much conflicting advice, how is anyone to know where the truth lies. Even the efforts published in our top medical journals fail to offer consistent guidance. Studies are often too small or too short, and there are many, many dropouts, which obscure accurate assessment.

Current Research

Two recent scientific surveys published in the *Journal of the American Medical Association* and in the *Annals of Internal Medicine* from Tufts and the University of Pennsylvania School of Medicine respectively, are typical. The first study done by Michael L. Dansinger and colleagues assessed adherence rates and effectiveness of the Atkins, Zone, Weight Watchers, and Ornish diets. One hundred and sixty participants were randomly assigned to one or another of these. After two months of maximum efforts, the participants selected their own levels of adherence.

At approximately one year, 50% of enrollees had dropped out. The weight losses at one year were 4 to 5 pounds and these were recorded only in the persons who stuck on the diet. Dansinger summarized that few stuck to their assigned diet. Weight loss on all diets was minimal, and that the amount of weight loss was associated specifically with the adherence but not with the diet type, indicating no particular advantage of any diet.

The other paper published in the *Annals of Internal Medicine* by Adam Tsai searched the Internet for major commercial weight-loss programs. They looked for the results of eDiets.com, Health Management Resources, Take Off Pounds Sensibly (TOPS), Optifast, and Weight Watchers. The conclusion was that these programs were associated with high costs, high dropout rates, and a high probability of regaining of the initial weight-loss. Weight loss was minimal. With the minor exception of one Weight Watchers trial, Tsai found little to support their use.

However, there's currently a study being run by my Stanford colleague, Christopher Gardner, that may offer some concrete guidance to us all. Gardner has four large groups of experimental diet subjects on the Atkins, Ornish, Zone, and South Beach diets. His groups are large enough, and so far the dropout rates are low. We await the results.

My Research

These questions take me back 40 years in my career when I received a large NIH research grant to study "The Effect of Diet on the Metabolism of Fat in Man."

We had a wonderful research program at the Lankenau Hospital in suburban Philadelphia. Nurses, nutritionists, exercise physiologists, bio-chemists were all searching for the *type* of food, the *amount* of food, and the *timing* of the food with regard to the nutritional profile for weight loss.

We had no trouble whatever locating volunteer subjects for our protocols. These individuals were men and women, lean and fat, some with diabetes. They became residents in our six bed ward in the Research Division. They were paid $10 per day, and in return, they allowed us to manipulate their diets and perform other radioisotope studies to measure different aspects of their metabolism. During the course of our study, we had nearly a hundred subjects who stayed with us for 3 to 24 months. For exercise, only casual walking around the ward was permitted.

Their diets were exclusively of the liquid formula type prepared daily in our research kitchen overseen by an expert dietitian. This guaranteed precision. We altered the constituents of the diet, maintaining a constant protein intake of 40g or 80g per day. The entire remainder of the daily calories was made up of either exclusively carbohydrate as cornstarch or fat as a vegetable oil emulsion, respectively. Taste was not an issue.

When the subject entered our unit, she was placed on a weight-maintaining number of mixed calories. If weight went up or down on the maintenance plan, we adjusted the calories accordingly so that the by the time the experimental diets were introduced we were confident that our subject was in a steady state and at a steady weight.

Fat Versus Carbs

After the initial baseline was established, the number of calories of the formula was reduced to 800 per day. When 40 grams of protein were provided, this yielded 160 calories, so the remaining 640 calories were given either entirely of carbohydrate or of fat. We alternated fats and carbohydrate intake, switching every three weeks. The results of the first 20 or so experiments revealed the rate of weight loss was absolutely identical regardless of whether the 640 calories came from fat or carbohydrate. When we doubled the protein to 80 grams per day, 320 calories of the 800, the same rate of a loss was observed as before as seen in Figure 15.

However, when we added five grams of salt daily to the formula feeding, a different pattern was observed. With salt in the diet when a subject went from the fat schedule to the carbohydrate schedule, a weight plateau was observed lasting a few days to a week. After this time, the rate of loss resumed at the former rate. When the subject alternated back to the fat protocol with no carbohydrate, there was a brisk and accelerated weight loss for several days until the original straight line was seen as shown in Figure 16.

Figure 15. **Isocaloric Fat/Carbohydrate Exchange and Weight Loss —Without Salt**

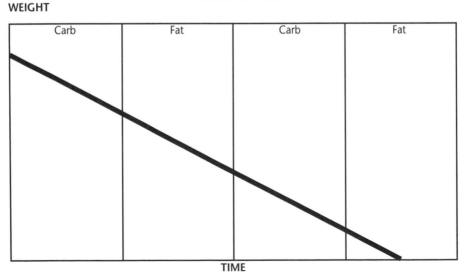

Figure 16. **Isocaloric Fat/Carbohydrate Exchange and Weight Loss —With Salt**

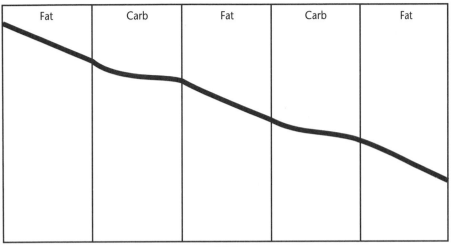

The explanation for this, of course, is the sodium or salt-retaining property of carbohydrate, or the water, losing property of fat. As fat is broken down into ketone bodies which are excreted in the urine, the kidney must neutralize the acidic nature of the ketone bodies and act like a diuretic. It loses sodium and its accompanying water to accomplish this.

This loss of water weight is the reason behind the usual pattern of rapid weight loss during the first several days of any diet. However, the body soon says "Whoa" within the next several days and the sodium and fluid loss is reversed. Weight loss ceases, despite fat loss continuing as before. The scale is unable to discriminate this fat loss from fluid retention. This pattern explains why the uninstructed dieter gives up in the second week because of a seeming lack of progress.

The take home message of these unambiguous and clear cut set of experiments is that apart from the fluid issue, carbohydrate and fat are precisely equivalent in their effect on the rate of weight loss. They are both lumps of coal in the furnace.

The Timing of Our Meals

A related set of experiments sought to establish whether the frequency of the feeding of the day's calories mattered to the rate of weight loss. This question was prompted by a set of papers from Edgar Gordon's group at the University of Wisconsin. These workers proposed that the many people's one meal a day gorging pattern results in an altered metabolic pattern that encourages obesity.

To investigate this proposition, we recruited six obese females into our study ward. After the weight stabilization, the calorie content of the mixed liquid formula diet was reduced to 600 calories per day, which was fed as 1, 3, or 9 feedings, (every two hours). The periods for each frequency diet were three weeks each. Careful daily weighing revealed that after an initial rapid weight loss secondary to fluid loss, the rate of loss was identical regardless of the frequency of the feeding. In other words, nibbling offered no advantage to gorging once a day. See Figure 17.

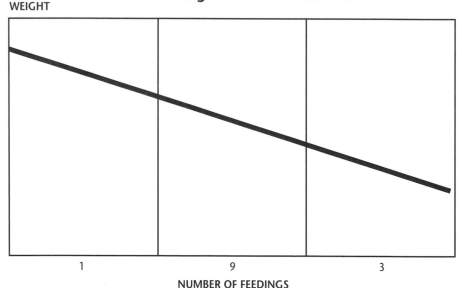

Figure 17. **Lack of Effect of Timing of Eating on Rate of Weight Loss—800 Calories**

WEIGHT

1   9   3

NUMBER OF FEEDINGS

How Many Calories Do We Need?

These experiments clearly established that the type and timing of the calories consumed did not matter. It followed naturally to establish the role of the *amount* of calories eaten on the rate of weight lost. The number of calories which a person needs is dependent upon their height, weight, age and gender. The taller and heavier and younger a person is, the higher will be their basal requirement. Males need more calories than females. Above this basal requirement of about one calorie per minute is the added need imposed by physical activity, which as mentioned above may be in extreme cases as high as 6,000 calories per day.

There are a number of tables available which accurately reflect the basal needs of different sizes, ages, and gender of persons. Any weight loss provoking diet will of necessity require eating fewer calories than the basal figure. What remains to be calculated then is how fast.

Three components provide these calories: carbohydrate, protein, and fat. A body has only a limited number of carbohydrate calories stored as sugar or starch, 800 to 1,200 calories. So this minimal storage cannot be used as an energy source for any prolonged period. Fat supplies 3,500 calories per pound. Dietary protein in our tissues is of course plentiful, but protein is our structure, so it is wiser not to rely on our flesh, our muscle, liver, kidneys for a calorie supply. And besides, protein is 80% hydrated in the body, and thus yields only 450 calories per pound. Even in starvation conditions, the body quickly shuts down its use of protein as an energy source. Our body is very, very smart.

Therefore of the body stores of carbohydrate, protein, and fat, only one is the appropriate energy source when dieting. Guess which one? Fat. It is admirably suited. It is light, as it is energetically dense. This is the major figure, the central number—3,500—on which the rate of weight gain and weight loss depends.

How to Drop the Pounds

For every overweight pound, a cumulative deficit of 3,500 calories needs be accrued in order to lose that pound. In order for an extra pound of fat to accumulate the person must take in 3,500 more calories than she needs. All primary care physicians are bedeviled by frequent encounters with patients who earnestly claim that they can't lose weight despite eating like a canary. Is it possible to maintain one's weight while eating a low calorie diet? We sought to answer that question.

We concluded that under our strict conditions there was no evidence whatsoever of anyone's ability to maintain weight while being underfed. A related observation is that there were no fat people in concentration camps. With the horrible starvation conditions that occurred there, any exceptions would have stood out vividly.

Calories Count

Having had this extensive experience in our research studies on the type and timing of calories, our group assessed our data. The accompanying figure represent a typical pattern in our study. These subjects were found to have a basal caloric need of 3,000 to 4,000 per day. After stabilization, the feedings were reduced to 800 calories per day, causing a 2,200 to 3,200 caloric deficit. By constructing a fraction of the deficit divided by 3,500 calories per pound, a projected rate of weight loss was created. The accompanying figure demonstrates a typical weight loss pattern in our study.

I published these results in the *Journal of the American Medical Association* April 1960 with the title "The Predictability of Weight Loss." The article has been abstracted, cited, and quoted hundreds of times. It has not, so far as I know, been repeated. It was expensive in time and money. Its conditions were severe, but the strict conditions under which this experiment was conducted validate its conclusions. CALORIES DO COUNT!

However, several important qualifications are necessary. Weight loss is absolutely predictable presuming that there are no major shifts in body water along the way. A 5-pound weight gain or loss from fluid retention may temporarily distort the expectation. Also, if a person embarks on a muscle building program while on a low calorie diet, the new muscle tissue built during resistance training may temporarily obscure the true weight loss being studied.

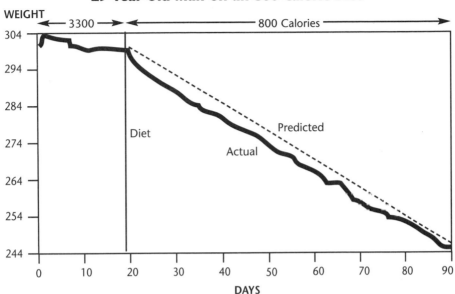

Figure 18. **Predicted and Actual Rate of Weight Loss of a 29-Year-Old Man on an 800 Calorie Diet**

A car drives the 400 miles from San Francisco to LA, getting 20 miles to the gallon. So it will require 20 gallons of gas to get there, 20 gallons of Union or Chevron or Texaco. The precise needs of our body are analogous. It's that simple.

But simplicity is hardly in evidence as we jump from diet to diet, each promising its unique advantages.

Do Diet Books Make Us Fat?

It seems that the more diet books published, the fatter we get. Which is cause and which is effect? No precise figures are available as the total number of diet books sold. It is estimated that their revenues approach $1 billion a year. Atkins has sold over 35 million copies by himself. These books promise no hunger, no pain, no guilt, exercise is rubbish, calories don't count, eat more, weigh less, eat right for your blood type, lose ten pounds in one week, lose fat here or there, wherever you desire, one absurd claim after another, each promising gratification and salvation.

Our gullibility quotient is seemingly boundless. Diet books span the range, the low-carb, and high fat formula of Atkins, to low fat, high carb of Ornish, with every conceivable variation in between.

With such a huge market of overweight people out there all seemingly with a huge appetite for books, the situation is right for the shrewd author to make a bundle. Focus groups would tell the ultimate diet book writer that the bestseller demands: 1) novelty, 2) simplicity, 3) celebrity, 4) cheap, 5) effective, and 6) long-term safety.

Armed with such market research, the prospective author might very well pen a book proposal for "The Britney Lard Diet" or "The Tiger Lettuce Diet." Britney and Tiger's diets would be novel, simple, cheap, and certainly effective, and the diet book writer need not worry about long-term safety. No one else seems to.

The point is that all diets work, provided that calories are cut. The diet books don't specifically acknowledge this fact in print, but every one of the fad diets is hypo-caloric: 1,200 to 1,700 calories a day of each one's chosen magic food.

They all exploit the fact that when food choice is limited to a few items, the body eventually recoils at the steady, boring restrictive regimen and, as a result, you eat less. There is no indication or evidence of long-term success of any single program. It's all about calories, but we knew that 40 years ago. The Britney Lard Diet, The Tiger Lettuce Diet, etc., etc. all work by cutting calories, but none has been proven to have any long-term advantage over any other.

The Kind of Carbs We Eat

A sub-theme of the carb/fat debate is the type of carb which we are talking about. Carbs vary greatly in their chemical nature from simple one-molecule substances, such as sugar, to multimolecular compounds, such as starch.

In the old days, the hunter-gatherer ate exclusively complex carbohydrate, simple sugars connected to form a chain. The enzymes which digest these have to work very hard to break this connection which then allows the simple sugars to be absorbed in the intestines. It is for this reason that the digestion of complex carbohydrates takes longer as compared to simple sugars, which require minimum effort to digest.

Complex carbohydrates were available in roots, leaves, and fruits—except when the hunter-gatherer wandered upon the honey of a bee's nest and a feast was declared. The scarcity of simple sugar as a dietary component continued until the 1700's, when the average Brit ate 3.5 pounds of sugar in a year. Now it is 150 pounds per year.

Sugar used to be a luxury item available to the wealthy aristocrats for their tea and crumpets. The opening up of the New World colonies—complete with vast new acreage for sugar cane fields—changed the carbohydrate landscape. Sugar consumption in England and Wales rose twenty-fold between 1632 and 1725. The price dropped. In 1942, the American Medical Association (AMA) expressed concern about the increased presence of soft drinks and candy. Feeling these sugary products constituted a health hazard, the AMA urged the limitation of their consumption. Since then, soft drink consumption has gone up sevenfold and overall sugar consumption has tripled.

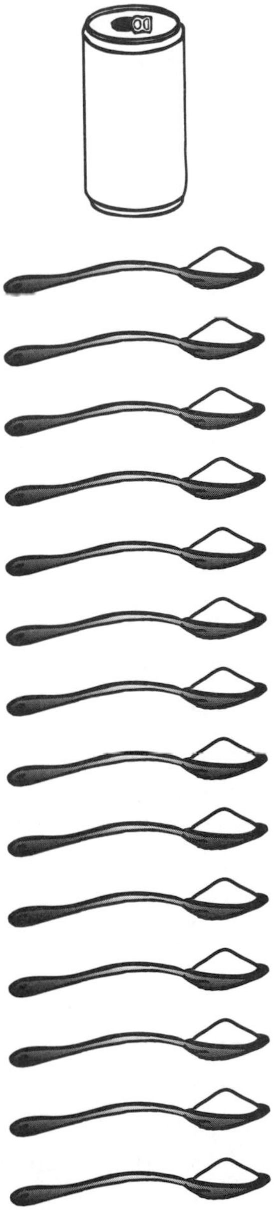

Mountains of Sugar

Twenty years ago teens drank twice as much milk as soda, the exact opposite of today's pattern.

Harvard researchers looked at the health experience of 51,603 women who were part of the Nurses Health

Figure 19

20 OZ. SODA =
14 TSP. OF SUGAR

Study. Women who consumed one or more sugary soft drinks per day had an 83% increased risk of Type 2 diabetes. An accompanying editorial pointed out that the higher sugar diet tends to be associated with other adverse health behaviors such as smoking and physical inactivity.

Without question, the switch from high-quality carbohydrate to low-quality sugar is a substantial contribution to obesity. Sugar is cheap, fast, and tasty. It is also a health risk.

Much of the current anti-carb rhetoric concerns itself with the ability of sugar to spark uneven insulin release, and thereby provoking erratic blood sugar levels. The glycemic index, a ranking of various foods based on their effect on blood sugar levels, attempts to rationalize this area, but this issue is more complex than the index indicates. After all, insulin doesn't cause obesity, calories do.

But the ease and rapidity and low cost of sugar in our world need to be constantly guarded against. In California, we are proud of our successful efforts to ban soda machines in the schools. This is a first meaningful step.

Slow Down

The Slow Food movement started in Rome in 1986 when Carlo Petrini was aghast when McDonald's opened a store on a famous piazza. The Slow Food idea is more than a diet; it is a way of life. It has advocates around the globe. They number close to 90,000 at the current time. It has many cultural implications, including support for local farmers and organic foods. Alice Waters of Chez Panisse fame and the Whole Food Stores are backers and enthusiasts. The symbol for Slow Food is the snail. They support the slow life.

Earlier, I demonstrated the timing of the day's calories didn't matter as long as the number of calories was low. Slow Food proposes that we tend to overeat because we eat so fast. The best-selling book, *Fast Food Nation* makes this point abundantly. Slow Food certainly has other psychosocial advantages. Think how far and between are the lingering family meals which define our character as a people. We all need to slow down, and if this is part of the strategy I'm all for it.

The exact opposite approach is tried by Fumio Kametsuzaki. This Tokyo gentleman heard about a fishpond which charged its anglers by the minute instead of by the catch. So he put this idea to test in a new restaurant featuring "all you can eat by the minute." An observer noted that the customers seemed to concentrate on being efficient chewers and swallowing rapidly. There's little talking in this restaurant, as people are determined to eat as much as quickly as possible. People wait in line in order to get in this restaurant. What is next?

Losing Weight Is not Impossible

If losing weight were easy, there wouldn't be so many diets and diet books out there. Breaking the cigarette and alcohol habits is even easier than losing weight, since with cigarettes and alcohol, total abstinence is a clear choice. This option obviously does not apply to food. The dieter is constantly confronted and contending with food. In many ways, it is easier to stop than to restrain. The statistics certainly aren't reassuring. The number of persons in the process of gaining weights is vast. The number of persons losing weight permanently is tiny. A variation on the old joke about smoking could be, "Who said losing weight was hard? I've done it a thousand times."

But losing weight is by no means impossible. It is crucial to recognize success, so that we confidently may say, "I think I can. I know I can. I did."

This success story is powerfully captured in an activity called the National Weight Control Registry. This important group was formed by Drs. Rena Wing from Brown, and Jim Hill of the University of Colorado in 1993. To qualify for the Registry, the applicant must have lost and maintained a weight loss of over 30 pounds for over one year.

To date, there are 4,800 enrollees, 60% are women, most are Caucasians, most are in their forties. Forty-six percent of the group was overweight as a child, 28% became obese as an adult, 46% had one obese parent, 27% had two obese parents. On average, these successful losers have lost 66 pounds, and have maintained this loss for 5 1/2 years. This is the gold standard. To accomplish this, 89% utilized both increased physical activity and diet in their programs. While 10% used diet alone, 1% used exercise exclusively. The group pursued every conceivable dietary pattern in their schedules. One-half of the group enrolled in some weight loss program, while the other half did it on their own.

The important conclusions from this optimistic survey were summarized by Wing and Hill:

- Most failures resulted from too much focus on diet and not enough on increased physical activity.
- Most programs focus more on losing weight than keeping it off. Losing weight strategies are different than those for keeping it off.
- Most persons maintained a low-fat diet with 1,300 to 1,500 calories per day. The diet pattern was consistent throughout the year.
- They all eat breakfast.
- They weigh themselves regularly.
- They walk a lot, 5.5 miles per day on average.

The crucial outcome of this study is that the participants universally report that their quality-of-life has greatly improved, and they are slim. You can keep weight off! This message is now being publicized in the latest food guide pyramid as one side of the pyramid is represented by exercise.

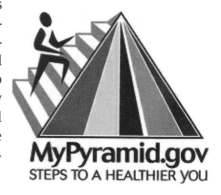

MyPyramid.gov
STEPS TO A HEALTHIER YOU

Why Do I Eat?

This simple question, along with its cousins, "What do I eat?" and "When do I eat?" seem like they should have simple answers. But even a brief reflection shows how complicated these three questions are.

You eat because you're hungry, right? But you may also eat when you're sad or glad, or even when you're angry. Certainly there are times I eat without being hungry, so it is clear that emotion plays a key role in our eating behavior.

The switches that control our eating are a hot scientific research area. When I was in medical school, my professor of physiology, Dr. John Brobeck, was one of the early researchers of the brain's appetite control centers. He found that there is a dual mechanism deep in the brain: when stimulated, one area causes intense hunger, while another when stimulated leads to an avoidance of food.

Signals

And new studies show it's not just our brain sending us signals about our nutritional needs. Different parts of the gastrointestinal tract send regular messages. Muscle and fat depots send signals, as do the endocrine glands, notably including the pancreas. The anatomical research is further enriched by discovery of a whole set of body chemicals, which also have double actions of stimulating and suppressing appetite.

Probably the first of these body appetite chemicals to be recognized and investigated was insulin. When a person or animal is given a shot of insulin, hunger is one of its first effects. This recognition led to a prominent theory concerning appetite control, called the glucostat theory. Insulin's action in lowering the blood sugar results in hunger, which is then relieved when the blood sugar goes back up. This led to the natural suggestion that the level of the blood sugar determined the degree of hunger which we experience. While this idea is still around, the situation is far more complicated.

Next was the lipostat theory, in which the amount of fat in our bodies was proposed to exert a negative control stimulus. The theory suggests that when we have an appropriate amount of lard around our bones it somehow serves to tell the mouth that enough is enough. This theory took on more weight with the discovery in 1994 of a hormone called leptin. This substance produced by the fat tissues was projected to be the chemical messenger that the adipose tissue sends to the brain to signal it to stop eating.

Leptin immediately generated huge commercial interest, with hopes that this represented the magic bullet of weight control. It seemed that salvation was close at hand. If we could put leptin in a pill form and give it to people who wanted to lose weight, the long-dreamed-for cure for obesity would be attained. Unfortunately, this was not to be. Despite several promising early reports, it was discovered that obese people had normal levels of leptin, which did not conform to theory. Hopes of giving leptin to overweight people to reduce their appetite have been pretty much abandoned.

Enter PYY or peptide YY, a molecule identified by endocrinologist, Stephen Bloom, at the Imperial College in London. He found that soon after the start of a meal, the cells of the lower intestine secrete a substance that he named PYY into the bloodstream. As its level builds up in the blood, it acts to slow down the action of the stomach and thereby creates the sensation of fullness, inhibiting further eating. In 2002, he published his results in the British journal, *Nature*. His work showed that PYY, when injected into the peritoneal cavity of rodents, and intravenously into people, would dampen hunger for at least 12 hours. Immediately, there was an outcry from other scientists disputing Bloom's claim and condemning his research. There is currently a staring match between the pro- and anti-Bloom findings. A recent article in *Science* stated that PYY is "too fickle" to provide a clue to the obesity remedy, and that there was still an immense amount of work to be done on the control of appetite.

Controlling Appetite

In any given year, the average person eats 750,000 to 1 million calories, and generally the body's fat content varies by only one to two pounds, which is 3,500 to 7,000 calories. This amazingly narrow control range occurs without our paying any attention. Our food intake device, our "appestat" if you will, provides ongoing information of when to eat and how much. It works in an amazingly efficient manner, with almost no messaging from us. The obesity epidemic is of course an alarm that this wonderful balance is distorted.

Psychologist Stanley Schachter theorized that a basic difference between lean and obese people is that lean folks eat when they listen to their hunger pangs. The obese, in contrast, eat more because of external cues from the environment, such as the clock.

To confirm this, he assembled a group of Columbia University students in a room where the clocks were altered. A bowl of crackers was placed before them and they were encouraged to help themselves. Schachter observed that the obese people ate when the clock said that it was dinnertime. The lean students were not affected by the clock setting, thereby proving Schachter's theory.

Al Stunkard, an old University of Pennsylvania professor of mine, showed that lean people feel hungry when their stomach contractions give notice. However, obese people's eating behaviors are not related to the gastric contraction pattern. Further, Schachter gave lean and obese individuals a taste test of ice cream of different qualities. The lean and obese didn't eat the poor quality product. All ate the high-quality product, but the obese group ate the lesser-quality mediocre products. He concluded his examples of the importance of external eating cues for overweight people, by constructing a scenario of a lean and obese person, passing a pastry shop or a McDonald's, shortly after having eaten. The lean person will walk briskly by. The obese person will succumb to the taste temptations which are only a few feet away.

Kafka observed, "There are two cardinal sins, impatience and laziness." We eat too fast, and move too slow. This simple and obvious reality is the perfect setting for our diabetes inferno.

6

Get Off the Couch and Save Your Life!

Exercise represents a higher rate of energy transfer. Exercise makes the engine run faster. You might query whether these higher RPM's don't result in a higher rate of wear and tear, and generation of more trash, such as the free radicals? Aren't you actually consuming the number of lifetime heart beats while running uphill when your pulse may reach 140 or higher? True enough, but as a result of the improved level of conditioning provided by hill running, the resting pulse rate falls to the 40s in contrast to the "norm" of 72 in unconditioned persons. So that the net number of heart beats in conditioned hill-running persons is less than the number of pulse beats in the sedentary individual.

Physical exercise is anabolic. It builds tissue. A weightlifter's biceps offers the best example. People who exercise have bigger arteries, stronger bones, and increased levels of brain growth factor. Exercise helps to reduce the incidence of some cancers. It restores the soul. Exercise raises the endorphin levels which increases pain tolerance and produces euphoria. Exercise helps the immune system and decreases the incidence of Alzheimer's disease. It is good for your sex life.

The benefits of physical exercise are many. The slackening of the movement of human beings is cause for general alarm, with Type 2 diabetes being among the most threatening.

Ten years or so ago, I was interviewed by Bryant Gumbel on the "Today Show." Midway through our upbeat chat, Bryant said, "Dr. Bortz, we don't have time to go into all your recommendations about the best diet. Of all your suggestions, what do you consider to be the most important regarding diet?"

I replied, "Move."

Biologically, We Move to Find Food

Movement is a defining part of biology, particularly animal life. Up and down the animal chain, the primary intent of this movement is to find food. We eat to move, and we move to eat. Or we used to, anyway. Contemporary humanity is the only species on earth which doesn't have to move to eat. We have uncoupled this tight relationship, an imbalance that is dangerous and flammable.

A central theme in biology is the "Principle of Least Effort," a law of profound evolutionary importance. It states that—winged, furry, scaled, big or little—any animal, when confronted by tasks such as food procurement or reproductive strategy, will select the means of accomplishing the task that requires the least amount of energy. You can't argue against that logic. When there's not that much to eat, it doesn't make sense to fly or run or swim around just for the fun of it. That unnecessary movement would create a need for even more calories.

Free Radicals

Coming along for the ride with physical exercise are the free radicals. Free radicals are like trash, the ashes which accrue simply by the chemical processes in the furnace which keeps us alive. Our body generates these free radical oxygen byproducts by the bushel. The theory is that free radicals are the price we pay to keep our engine moving. (By the way, the nasty free radicals are also widely given credit as the principal agents responsible for aging.)

The faster we run our engine, the more free radicals generated. So physical exercise revs up the revolutions in our engine, causing the formation of more free radicals. But that same exercise also increases the production of crucial enzymes catalase, glutathione reductase, and superoxide dismutase. These enzymes very efficiently destroy the free radicals almost as quickly as they are formed. On balance, therefore, exercise results in a net reduction of free radicals—not by reducing their production, but by increasing their destruction, stories much like the heartbeats.

Free radicals are increasingly thought to contribute to cell death. They are incriminated in the destruction of the beta cells in Type 1 and in advanced Type 2. Exercise helps to offset their mischief and retards cell death.

Being Lazy or Conserving Energy?

All animals economize their movement to just what is necessary. Our hunter-gatherer and farmer ancestors moved only as much they needed to. However, this amount was still far in excess of that required to stave off obesity.

Contemporary mankind flaunts this imperative. We have electric golf carts, battery driven toothbrushes, electric carving knives, and remote control TV channel changers all designed to save our energy. I envision high rise buildings stuffed with engineers and PR people all working feverishly to design a product that will spare us from having to move at all. Given the choice to move less, we move less. The conservation of energy is etched into our biology.

My Inner Bushman

I conjure up the following scenario as my inspiration to run my annual marathon, which I have done the last 35 years. At the starting line in Boston, I envision myself needing to track a bush buck for 26 miles. If successful, my survival for another year is assured.

Exercise is good for you—for every part of you, from your hairline to your toes. Everybody needs it. We have a minimum daily requirement (MDR) for vitamins, calcium, calories, how about an MDR for exercise? The Centers for Disease Control and the

American College of Sports Medicine both proclaim that one half hour of moderate physical intensity exercise on most days of the week is our basic need. Evidence suggests that more is better.

Fit and Fat

Physical activity has a long list of favorable benefits beyond its carbohydrate use facilitating function. Exercise physiologist Steve Blair of the Cooper Aerobics Institute has extensively written on the topic "Fit and Fat." He finds that fat persons who are fit are at about the same health risks as lean persons who are unfit. Restated, physical fitness covers up some of the calamities which being overweight causes. The implications of this observation are obviously of great importance when considering the diabetes inferno, and what strategies can be evolved to confront it.

How Do We Measure Exercise?

Is there a way to measure the amount of exercise we get? One scientific method is to measure the amount of oxygen used during a particular activity. The quantity consumed provides a concise calculation of the amount of work that has been performed. Another measurement method is to assay the calories that are expended while doing a task.

A further measuring tool which is being increasingly referred to is "met"—short for metabolic equivalent. One met is defined as the amount of energy or exercise which you use at rest. You can't go lower than that. Drs. Barbara Ainsworth and Bill Haskell have developed a table which is widely used to figure out how much exercise is being performed. Using this met intensity value of exercise multiplied by the amount of time which it is being pursued leads to a numerical value expressed in met hours. Lying in bed for one hour is one met hour. Walking for one hour is three met hours. Running for one hour is eight met hours.

Count Your Steps

In an effort to provide a measurement tool that is simpler and more practical, Dr. Jim Hill of the University of Colorado School of Medicine suggests counting the number of steps as an alternative method of gauging the amount of exercise. Three advantages of using steps: first is the availability of cheap and reasonably reliable pedometers. Second, it addresses the most common form of exercise: walking. And third, the number of steps allows an entire day's activity to be estimated and so is not merely confined to valuing an interval of exercise. Oxygen consumption, calories, mets, and steps are all strategies which we use to try to give understanding of the amount of physical activity that a person is pursuing.

To get a sense of how all of these measurements address the same thing let's look at the energy involved in walking.

$$1 \text{ hour walking} = 6,000 \text{ steps}$$
$$= 3 \text{ met hours} = 180 \text{ calories}$$
$$= 1/20 \text{ pound of fat/day}$$

Or

$$10,000 \text{ steps} = 300 \text{ calories}$$
$$= 1/12 \text{ pound of fat/day}$$

On average, people gain two pounds of fat per year. This equals 7,000 additional calories. Seven thousand calories per year breaks down to 20 calories per day, or an additional 660 extra steps per day. In other words, walk a bit more and you needn't gain that extra two pounds each and every year. This is a battle that can be won!

Buck the Trend: Take More Steps, Not Fewer

Some highly-trained individuals can increase their level of energy expenditure up to 20 times their basal level, but this intensity can be only briefly sustained. The largest sustained exercise load documented is during the Tour de France bicycle race, two weeks of extremely strenuous exercise in which on average the riders expend 6,000 calories per day, approximately five times their basal energy expenditure. In order to raise the bar to this level, a great deal of physical conditioning is required. An unfit person can only double his basal exercise level.

So knowing the range of what is possible for each of us, we then should ask ourselves how much are we doing? How much should we do?

An interesting study came out of Australia four years ago. Seven male actors were hired to impersonate Australian settlers in the good old days, 150 years ago, before modern technology. The settlers/actors were observed for one week, with their activity levels carefully noted. The observation concluded that the "settlers" were 2.3 times more active than today's office workers.—the equivalent of walking ten more miles per day. Present day hunter-gatherers, on average move 11.5 miles per day.

Ninety-nine percent of people take the escalator and elevator rather than stairs. For every two hours spent watching TV each day, your obesity risk goes up 23% and risk of Type 2 diabetes increases by 14%. Men watch 29 hours per week. Women watch 34 hours. A story in the *National Geographic* recorded that in 1960, 62% of us drove to work, 10% walked, and 14% took public transportation. In 2000, 90% drove to work, 3% walked, and 6% took public transportation. Back in Mexico, the Pima Indians used 520 more calories per day than they did after their move to Phoenix. Members of an order of Amish farmers in Canada take 18,925 steps per day, versus the 2,000 to 3,000 steps taken per day in the average urban life style.

Move to Lose

Even a casual reflection reveals how the landscape of America has changed from farm to shopping mall. Asphalt has replaced orchards. Subdivisions have replaced city neighborhoods. Once we were a nation of villages, towns, and a few cities. Flying at night above America reveals lights everywhere. Los Angeles is the prototype of the American big-city, with little or no dark places left, but hundreds of acres of freeways.

The automobile was the spark of the landscape revolution. People fled to the suburbs by the tens of millions. City centers are ghostlike at night, as most metropolitan areas. Citizens are asleep or watching TV in their remote retreats.

Figure 20.

OPPORTUNITIES TO BURN CALORIES ...	CALORIES	... AND WHAT WE DO INSTEAD	CALORIES
Getting off couch to change TV station	3	Use remote	0.6
Mowing the lawn by hand	500/hr	Electric lawn mower	180/hr
		Lawn service	0
Walking a flight of stairs	5	Taking the escalator/elevator	0.3
Playing outside for 4 hours	900	Watching TV	350
30 minutes of ironing	35	Taking clothes to the cleaners	0
Chopping vegetables for 15 minutes	10.3	Buying already cut vegetables	0
Bicycling for 20 minutes	200	Riding in a car	0
Cleaning for 1 hour	240	Hiring someone to clean	0
Raking leaves	150	Leaf blower	100
Manually opening the garage door twice a day	23	Garage door opener	0.25
Getting up and answering the phone and standing for three ten-minute conversations	20	Using the portable phone while lying on the couch for 30 minutes	4
Dancing for 30 minutes	150	Sitting watching dancing	25
Parking at far end of parking garage and walking for 3 minutes	24	Parking near the door with a 10-second walk	0.5
Scrubbing floors for 1 hour	440	Hire someone to wash floors	0

Commuting to work is now standard. Many people spend 20% of their waking hours driving to and from work. The average American mother spends over one hour every day in her car. Between 1982 and 1997, the average Atlanta resident doubled his driving commuting distance.

There is a nearly complete lack of large scale, longitudinal, quantitative population studies on the amount of physical activity which people have pursued through the years. One such study was published recently and included data from a large group of Swedish men from the years 1932 to 1997. Thirty-three thousand four hundred and sixty-seven men were questioned about their total physical activity and Figure 21 is derived from these studies. The solid line represents the actual amounts expressed as met hours per day through 1997. The dotted lines from 1997 onward are a reasonable extrapolation. If one continues the extrapolation of the available data, to the year 2130 the total daily physical activity will reach 24 mets per day, which is equivalent to lying in bed. Such extrapolation is similar to the one suggested by Professor J. P. Foreyt for the future prevalence of obesity in America. His figure indicated that in 2050 there will only be one lean person left in all of America. And it seems that he or she will likely still be in bed. Is this where we are headed?

Figure 21. **Decline in Physical Activity over Time**

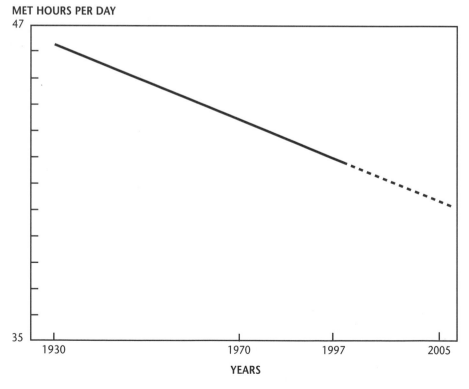

America is the least active country on earth. Blame Henry Ford, but we surely do love our cars. The car cult is deeply embedded in our value system. Why walk when I can drive? Our habitat is not leg friendly.

With leadership from CDC and the Robert Wood Johnson Foundation, there's a brighter beam being thrown on urban planning. Sidewalks, bike lanes, nearness to parks and trails are all encouraged to promote leg-friendly environments.

What if our legs withered and vanished in an evolutionary development due to urban sprawl? Like the wings of the dodo bird who no longer had to fly to live, have our legs lost their functional utility? It seems the wheel has replaced them, just as keyboards and switches have replaced our arms.

Obesity and Lack of Exercise

The debate over which element is the prime contributor to obesity goes on. Some advocates concentrate on inactivity as the principal contributor. Others advocate overeating. The answer lies in between. Darius Lakdawalla at the National Bureau of Economic Research estimates that 65% of the increase in obesity is tied to decreased calorie needs due to mechanization.

The Important Work of Jean Mayer

Jean Mayer was a preeminent nutritionist and authority on obesity in all its manifestations. During his time at Harvard, he published two studies that I feel are among the most important ever done with regard to weight control. The first was published in the *American Journal of Physiology*. The main results are depicted in Figure 22.

The study lasted 45 days. In it, the physical activity of the rats was perfectly regulated so that they ate precisely the appropriate amount of food to sustain body weight while engaging in physical exercise, running. However, when the rats were encouraged to increase their run to over six hours a day, the exercise became stressful. Their appetite and weight decreased.

Figure 22. **Weight, Calorie Intake and Physical Activity of Rats**

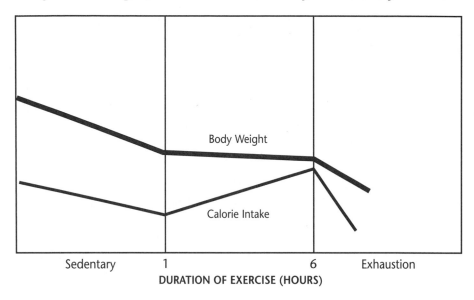

The crucial part of the experiment is presented at the other side of the graph. As the rats were prevented from exercise, their calorie intake increased to the amount they consumed while running for 2 hours. Consequently, they gained weight. This finding says to me that the brain appetite center in a rat's hypothalamus is tightly keyed to the exercise demands until the activity is withdrawn. The hypothalamus does not receive a negative signal and weight gain ensues.

Mayer and colleagues visited a mill in West Bengal, near Calcutta. They sought out a work site with workers who exhibited a wide range of physical activities in their job performance. Figure 23 shows the impact of job-related physical activity on body weight and food intake.

Those workers who exerted 2,500 calories of activity or more per day maintained a normal weight. Their sedentary companions ate more and gained 30 lbs. as the result of the double whammy of more calories in and fewer calories out. See Figure 23.

Mayer filmed 13- to 17-year-old girls at a Cape Cod summer camp. The obese girls' weight averaged 176 pounds, the lean girls' 118 pounds. He performed timed motion studies of these 108 stu-

Figure 23. **Weight, Calorie Intake and Physical Activity of Indian Mill Workers**

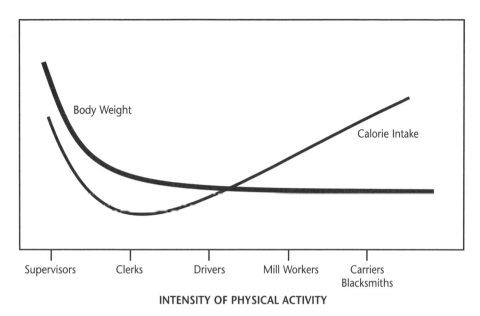

dents, observing that the obese girls were inactive for 77% of the time when they were playing tennis, and lean girls were inactive for only 56%. During volleyball, the figures were 90% versus 69%. In yet another study, he looked at 28 obese and 28 non-obese high school girls. The obese girls ate 1,900 calories per day, the lean girls 2,700.The obese girls were active only four hours per week, versus 11 hours per week for the lean proving the significance of physical activity in weight management.

Data presented by the National Bureau of Economic Research indicates that workers who spend their careers in a sedentary job have a Body Mass Index that is 3.3 units higher than those who are in active jobs. This difference is equivalent to the weight that has been gained across the population during the last 100 years.

The Sumo Story

This story arises from a 1,500 year old cultural tradition in Japan. Sumo wrestlers—those huge men in diapers—have been introduced to us via TV. Sumo wrestling matches are a strange sight, somewhere between a dance form and professional wrestling. Much of these highly, ritualized events take place before the match outside the ring, as the actual hand combat is short and abrupt. Seven seconds is the average duration of a bout.

The encounter commences with slapping of thighs, stomping of feet to expel demons, throwing of salt to purify the ring and the glowering. The gesturing has evolved from ancient Shinto rituals. Eventually, one wrestler rushes at the other, followed by a brief tussle as each sumo strives to eject the other from the ring.

These fellows make professional football linemen look like school kids. They may weigh in excess of 600 pounds. The great Hawaiian wrestler Konishiki once weighed in at 690. Weight provides a big competitive advantage

Their daily routine is interesting. They arise at 6 am, often in a shared dormitory, and then take part in a strenuous five-hour workout, sometimes including 500 leg lifts before the first of two huge meals. One account reported 70 pieces of sushi and mega bottles of beer consumed at one setting. Five thousand calories is the usual daily intake. Immense amounts of meat, rice, with liberal amounts of alcoholic beverages thrown in, just to wash it all down.

Their extraordinary bulk prompts a major health interest. Unfortunately, there is no systematic survey of their medical experiences, but many anecdotal reports exist. First, their longevity is short; 60 years of age is a long life for them. Most retire when they are still in their twenties because of precocious foot and knee arthritis. In the only reference I found, there is a 5.2% incidence of diabetes among Sumo wrestlers. Though higher than non-sumo Japanese men, it is still below what might be predicted for people of such immense size. Perhaps their level of physical activity confers a protective effect.

Children and Inactivity: Turn Off the Television

Recent statistics on the health of our children are even more startling than those of the adults. There was a tenfold increase in Type 2 diabetes in children from 1982 to 1994. For them, the inactivity /obesity /diabetes linkage is crucial. Children in 1955 played and used 900 calories in 4 hours, today children use 350 calories watching TV. Stanford colleague and noted childhood obesity expert Tom Robinson figures 25% of waking hours are spent watching TV, which is bad enough, but 20% of the daily calories are consumed while sitting in front of the TV screen. Children burn 550 less calories a day then children of 50 years ago. Is it any wonder we have an obesity problem among our youth?

That Goes for Grownups, Too!

A recent Mayo Clinic time motion study finds that obese people spend 571 minutes per day sitting and 373 standing during the entire day. The corresponding numbers for the lean group were 407 minutes sitting and 506 minutes on their feet. The couch potato image is confirmed. If the obese individuals substituted 164 minutes of their sitting time into standing, this would add 352 more calories expended per day to their balance sheet. Similarly, a walk to and from work would contribute 150 calories per day to this requirement.

The Benefits of Fidgeting

Separate and distinct from the calorie equivalent provided by physical activity of various sorts is a fascinating feature termed "fidgeting." Over 50 years ago, noted nutrition expert E. M. Widdowson of Cambridge, England described fidgeting as an important and usually overlooked component of calorie disposal. This work was picked up by Erik Ravussin when he was with NIH in Phoenix. It is now being surveyed by James Levine at the Mayo Clinic. Anywhere from 100–700 calories per day may be accounted for merely by the energy demands imposed by fidgeting. This jumpiness is in turn correlated with the overall setting of the autonomic nervous system and its adrenaline cells. This finding partially explains why some people seem to be able to eat more than others due to their high fidgeting quota. It is hard to imagine prescribing a dose of fidgeting for overweight persons. But this is at least a hypothetical strategy.

Every survey indicates that we are moving less and less. Less than 40% of Americans are even minimally physically active, this inactivity plays no age favorites. Kids and oldsters sit too much. I spent much of my professional career asserting that many of the changes including the upward trend in diabetes incidence that is commonly attributed to aging per se is in reality due to the increased sitting time that older people defer to. *Use it or lose it* is a powerful aphorism.

The Evidence Is In

Numerous large observational studies address the inactivity/obesity/diabetes/mortality axes. An eight year review of 70,000 nurses revealed 1,419 new cases of diabetes. Physically fit nurses had half the incidence of diabetes as the physically unfit. A Cooper Aerobic Center study showed that unfit men were four times as likely to become diabetic than fit men over 14 years. A survey of 34,257 women in Minnesota revealed that "any" amount of physical activity lowered the incidence of new diabetes by 30%. A study in Malmo, Sweden reviewed the life history of a group of people with pre-diabetes and found that an exercise intervention lowered their mortality to that of persons who were not pre-diabetic. Exercise "cured" pre-diabetes, at least as far as mortality was concerned.

Going to bed for 72 hours lowers glucose utilization by 50%. The incidence of diabetes is substantially increased after spinal cord injury or any misadventure that hinders mobility.

These results consistently demonstrate the great benefit of physical activity. Those who make public policy should place a much higher priority on encouraging physical activity.

Small Steps Big Rewards

The next step in ownership is to set reasonable expectations. If you have not done any form of physical activity in 20 years, don't try walking a mile as you begin your exercise plan. The Small Steps Big Rewards plan published by the National Diabetes Education Program suggests setting short-term goals that guarantee success. You can then build on these small successes. If you are eating 3 cups of pasta as a serving, ½ cup isn't going to cut it. Reducing your portion size to 2 cups may be a more realistic and achievable goal. And you are more likely to continue on your weight loss program.

In order to change behavior, you need to stay motivated. It is important for you to identify what it is that will keep you on track—whether it is the desire to see your children grow up and marry, or to spend time with grandchildren, or to feel well enough after your retire to see all those exciting places that exist around the world. Whatever that special something is, determine what will provide you with the motivation to keep going when the going gets rough.

Support of family and friends is crucial. That does not mean family members can be "diabetes police" but rather they can be positive and supportive of your efforts. Something as simple as going encouraging an early morning or evening stroll each day, or making sure the refrigerator and pantry are filled with healthy food choices are wonderfully loving actions of someone who lives with and loves a diabetic. Hey, if the wrong foods aren't available, your temptations will be lessened.

Further, if you have diabetes, your family is at risk, so they should be eating the right foods as well. That is also true as far as their need for a healthy lifestyle. Engaging the entire family in a plan to practice healthy behaviors is important. Parents should act as role models for their children. Likes and dislikes are developed at an early age. If children see parents engaging in physical activity as part of their daily routine, they are much more likely to develop similar, healthy habits.

7

The Financial Ravages of the Diabetes Inferno

In April 2005, the Commerce Department reported that America's net income went down for the first time in over half a century. We are not making less money, but our expenses, in large part due to the surge in health care costs, are rising faster than our productivity.

Surging Numbers

The surging numbers of diabetes cases are finally getting attention. Not only magazine editors, but health insurers, governmental policymakers, hospitals, pharmaceutical companies, everyone is being singed in major ways by the health consequences of diabetes. More than just a physical burn, the fire exacts a devastating economic cost.

The associated financial burdens will threaten national treasuries. From 1997 to 2002, costs attributable to diabetes doubled from 68 to 132 billion dollars in America alone.

Diabetes Price List

How much does diabetes cost? How can what we lose be defined: more than a nuisance, it results in anxiety, discomfort, lost wages, disability expenses, doctor's visits, drug costs, hospital bills. Is there a way to quantify the costs of this dreadful disease?

Think about your health as your checking account. As such, it is an important asset in your life like your home equity or your shares of General Electric or your car. But your health is a vastly more important asset than all those material possessions. It is no less real than they are, but you just don't stop to consider your health as a tangible treasure of your life. It is.

Health Account

To continue the metaphor of health as wealth, it is important to realize that your health has a wide surplus of safety. Health has much redundancy built into it, just like a space capsule. Consider the paired organs of your body. You have two eyes, two ears, two lungs, two kidneys, two testicles or ovaries, and you can lose one of them, one eye, ear, lung, and kidney or sex gland and still get by without seeming a problem. You can see adequately with one eye, hear okay with one ear, run a marathon with only one lung, excrete enough waste with one kidney, or overpopulate the world with one testicle. This means that you can surrender 50% of your health account without functional distress. You can even give away another 10% with no problem. Lose another 10%, dropping down to 30% of starting allotment, and symptoms start. Shortness of breath, weakness, toxicity, blurred vision, or dulled hearing, or diabetes. The alert is sounded. Another 10% loss down to 20% of full competency, and you are legally blind, or deaf, infertile, or dead.

Overdraft Notice

So it is in the 20% to 30% range where virtually the entirety of our nation's $1.8 trillion annual medical expense occurs: $4 billion each day, $3 million each minute, $50,000 each second is spent on hospitals, surgery, technology, and pharmacy. This amount is spent in the effort to get out of the red and into the black part of the health ledger sheet.

When you have $200,000 in your health account, you can be a big spender. But if you only have a buck and a half in the bank, you better watch your pennies. The problem is, of course, most of us have a much firmer fix on how much is in our checking accounts than in our health accounts. Also, many figure that this issue is really not important to worry about because if an overdraft or bankruptcy notice appears, you can always seek out your friendly family practitioner or pharmacist, and he or she will bail you out.

Don't count on it. This is one of the big unspoken fallacies. When the red ink appears in an empty health account, the medical system is limited in its restorative capabilities.

Health Assets

What drains your health assets? Genes, external agency, internal agency, and aging. With these separate and distinct categories the whole of a person's life health history can be described.

These are more easily understood if a car analogy is invoked. A car's health depends on design, accidents, maintenance and how old it is—same for you. If you are a lemon, a bad seed or chromosomal mismatch, or insist on running into things, or put bad fuel in your tank, or run your machine too hard or not hard enough, then the car, like you, will not have the chance to grow old.

Genes

Genes, our design, are important, but they probably represent not more than 15% of your total health profile. Most problems caused by genes are notable in the early part of life. Heredity is a relatively minor contributor to the diabetes inferno.

Accidents

Accidents happen. That's what we call an external agency; infections, injury, malignancies, toxins are part of life. For some people, they are catastrophic and maybe fatal, more so in the past. Today, for most of us, accidents result in a series of pulled tendons, broken ribs secondary to a hostile encounter with a big tree limb, a busted baseball finger, and the like.

I include Type 1 diabetes in my category of health expenditures due to external agency. These conditions are episodic, caused by something from the outside and don't really have anything to do with personal behavior in their causation. The affected person is an innocent bystander who suddenly gets an overdraft notice as 70% to 80% of the beta cell reserve is lost. Such a loss of reserve function in kids usually happens very abruptly, dropping from 100% to 20% to 30% within a week or two.

This is a fairly accurate analogy between the health asset represented by the full account of beta cells and insulin and Type 1 diabetes. The analogy is made more complex, however by the natural healing, recovery function of the body and all its parts. While it is accurate to depict beta cell and insulin loss as a sudden destruction, at the same time the tissues of the body are resisting the damage and trying to heal. This is where an analogy to a car breaks down. A car can't heal its problems on its own. The body has awesome reparative capacity.

Such reparative capacity, with regard to Type 1 diabetes may be the explanation behind the "diabetes honeymoon" phenomenon where the diabetic process in its early stages seems to fluctuate.

Maintenance

This likening of Type 1 diabetes to an accident or a problem of external agency is different from the story of Type 2. Instead of the health account, beta cell reserve, being debited by a sudden huge expense it is debited incrementally, a penny at a time. This depletion of cell reserve is so insidious that by the time the overdraft slip arrives, much collateral damage has already occurred. Type 2 diabetes is a problem of poor maintenance, a problem of disordered internal agency, both with regard to the fuel component, and also how hard the machine is run. Initially, in its course, the beta cells and insulin are intact, and only after years of overspending does the overdraft note arrive.

Age

Tom Perls, from the important Harvard Centenarian Study, surveyed 425 persons ranging from 97 to 119. His group categorizes these exceptional persons into three groups, which they entitled Survivors, Delayers, and Escapers. The Survivors are those who encountered a major illness before age 80 and still lived to celebrate their 100th birthday. Of the group, 24% of the men and 43% of the women were Survivors. Delayers were those who developed an illness after the age of 80, but still made 100. Forty four percent of men and 42% of women fit this profile. The Escapers were the 32% of men and 15% of the women, who sailed through ten decades of life without encountering any major illness bumps along the way.

You can analyze this portrait of being 100 a variety of ways. The interpretation I favor is that it's always wonderful to avoid and escape trouble along life's route, but that even if trouble is encountered, survived and delayed along the way, life clings to life.

Is it even possible for a person with diabetes to make it to 100? Having read the first part of the book, you already know the answer to the question. Even for a child with diabetes, living to 100 is a possible goal if life is lived with "guts and smarts." The inherent vigor and spirit of the human organism is a miracle. We have the responsibility to cherish life. We must avoid self-destructive tendencies, and constantly protect our health asset. It is never too late to embrace this reality, but it is always too soon to abandon it or ignore it.

Thinking of your health and your pancreas in financial terms is a new concept that in my view is important in order to create a new and different context of the Diabetes Danger. This new way of thinking may encourage us to conceive of a comprehensive remedial strategy. Having established the qualitative parameters of your health account leads directly to the effort to apply dollar amounts to some of these aspects.

How Much is a Life Worth?

Have you ever stopped to ask yourself this basic, obviously important and defining question? Almost no one has. Answers to this probing question may find a reference site in the literature of economics and personal injury. But from what I've generally understood, the value of a human life is roughly gauged as three million dollars.

Does this make any sense? The analysts come up with such a figure by calculating the production of that life, the 50 years of productive labor times $60,000 per year, or some other combination of duration and income per unit time. Such calculation yields this crude estimate of $3 million per life.

Another derivation of the $3 million per life value is to divide the United States' Gross National Product (GNP) of $10 trillion by this country's population (300,000,000), yielding 3 million per life again.

Are all lives worth the same? Can lives have a dollar value put on them at all? The $3 million price tag placed on the value of one life is clearly a crude estimate, but it is nonetheless a useful actuarial figure to reference when calculating some of the costs of the diabetes inferno.

But before I discuss the financial costs of diabetes, the personal costs must be first addressed. The individual stories of challenge and heartache and anger and daily distresses of a hundred different types cannot be counted. No dollar figure can remotely approach the individual burdens which diabetes imposes.

I divide the personal costs into the short-term and long-term. The short-term personal costs which diabetes charges the afflicted person involve the moment-to-moment awareness and responses which are inherent in the disease. Someone estimated that the average person with diabetes thinks about her disease approximately once every 15 minutes of the waking day. Such preoccupation with anything is a major cost by itself, but then an accounting must be made of what this awareness involves. "What did I eat? When did I eat? When will I eat? What should I eat? What is my blood sugar? How much exercise will I get in? What effect will it have on my blood sugar and my treatment schedule?" Take these questions and multiply them by a hundred and a daily roster of the diabetic person's consciousness is sampled.

Burying your head in the sand like an ostrich has an immense appeal to all of us when confronted by huge tasks. For diabetics, this is not an alternative. It is a stern taskmaster 24/7/365.

The issues don't go away. Neglect is sinister.

Long Term Costs

Halfway consciousness imposes a tax on future health. Even short-term expediency or inattention is full of future peril. No disease—from AIDS to leprosy to cancer, whatever dread disease you care to nominate—has a more dreadful complication list than diabetes. The list is long, varied, and scary: heart failure, strokes, amputations, nerve pain, impotency, kidney disease, intestinal disturbance, depression, and skin problems. No body system, or body cell is immunized from the cruelty of diabetes.

Again, how can a person possibly put a price tag on this misery? Adding the costs of short-term daily personal burden to the pervasive long-term costs of complications creates a ledger that overflows with red ink.

Life Quality Costs

Putting the short-term and long-term personal costs of diabetes into a single parameter is impossible. But major economists, notably Richard Zechauser of Harvard, have championed the effort to mix quantity and quality together by generating a term with the acronym of QALY: quality adjusted life year. This term addresses the issue of the diminished quality-of-life imposed by a certain condition. A number emerges by asking a large group of healthy people how they would rate the quality of a life which is burdened by diabetes, for example, as compared to that life which does not carry that diagnosis and the baggage that goes with it. The general figure that is generated for diabetes is 0.75.

Said another way, the overall quality of one year of life with diabetes is only 75% of the value of one without. This overall estimate is further extended by additional qualifying burdens of those miserable conditions associated with diabetes. What is the quality of life, the QALY, for a person with diabetes with an amputation, or blind, or on dialysis three times per week with kidney failure, or congestive heart failure?

These quantitative estimates address only the subjective quality of the individual's life. Separate and beyond the subjective estimates are the actual dollar amounts which are imposed by the different conditions. The ideal life of course is one that is full of quality and lived as long as possible.

Many indicators assert that 100 years represents the average human lifetime potential. Few reach that number, even fewer diabetics. But it is not the quantity of the years which are of greatest concern, but the quality of those years. If the last years of life are lived with the burden of one or more of the serious complications that diabetes courts, the QALY is much lower.

But even worse, since we know that virtually the entirety of the complications are preventable, the responsibility of minimizing the morbidity, disability, and QALY figures is a paramount task for society and all its citizens. Presently, we are doing a miserable job of accepting this responsibility.

Every Day, More Dollars for Diabetes

The Centers for Disease Control and American Diabetes Association both report that the medical costs attributable to diabetes in 2002 were a staggering $132 billion. This huge figure is made even more unsettling when you consider that's a full 30% higher than just five years before.

At a more individual level, the ADA reports the person without diabetes had an average annual medical care cost of $3,000. In contrast, a diabetic had an average annual medical care cost of $14,000, $11,000 for person per year more! Overall, the health care costs of diabetics are four to five times more than persons who do not have this diagnosis.

If one in three babies and one in two Hispanic newborns are destined to become diabetic, you can calculate the bankrupting effect of these charges.

Of the gross figure of $132 billion for 2002, $92 billion were accounted for by what are termed "direct" medical costs, $40 billion come from "in-direct" costs which are disability, work and productivity losses, and premature mortality.

Of the $92 billion direct costs, $23 billion arise from diabetes care expense, $25 billion from chronic disease diabetes related complications, and $44 billion attributable to general medical conditions. Forty billion dollars was secondary to inpatient hospital charges, (16.9 million days), and $14 billion from nursing home charges secondary to diabetes.

There were 63 million doctor office visits related to diabetes in 2002.

Twelve billion dollars in cost figures come from drug and insulin use, $7.5 billion from oral agents and $3.9 billion from insulin.

There is an age component to these charges, as 52% of all charges—$48 billion of the direct costs—are from persons over 65 years of age.

A composite estimate of the value of lives lost to diabetes can be derived from the 186,000 deaths in 2002 directly attributable to diabetes (a number that is certainly an underestimate), times $117,000 lost earnings per life lost, yielding a figure of $21.7 billion.

Additionally, in 2002 it is estimated that there were 88 million days of work lost to the disability associated with diabetes and 176,000 cases of permanent disability incurred which cost $8 billion. The average daily wage figure of $160 per day yields $15.5 billion lost to productivity waste.

It is critical to recognize that these are figures derived from 2002. While the most recent available, they are already outdated. It can be confidently predicted that all of these charges will be much, much higher.

So the costs of diabetes, personal, organizational, national are staggering and getting worse.

What can we do?

It is instructive to try to estimate what can be done via preventive effort to offset these charges. With regard to obesity roughly costing 200 billion dollars in 2005: If we assume that the entirety of the 200 billion-dollar cost secondary to obesity is due to physical inactivity, one can derive the following estimate: $200 billion per year for 130 million overweight Americans yields $1,500 cost per overweight person per year.

Below, the numbers may get confusing, but follow closely and you will see how just adding a few daily steps saves money. They may also possibly save your life!

The average amount of excess weight an overweight person has is 25 pounds. Take the $1,500 cost per person per year cited above, divide it by 25 pounds is $60 per pound. One pound equals 3,500 calories, which equals 10 hours walking which equals 60,000 steps. 6,000 pennies divided by 60,000 steps yields a value of ten steps. So we can conclude that taking ten steps saves one cent in obesity costs.

If, however, we acknowledge that physical inactivity is only partially responsible for the obesity costs as quantified by Darius Lakdawalla and Tomas Philipson from the National Bureau of Economic Research, it follows that 200 billion dollars multiplied by 60% = 120 billion dollars secondary to inactivity, and 80 billion dollars secondary to caloric excess. Therefore, if inactivity alone accounts for 120 billion dollars, 18 steps saves one cent in obesity costs.

Steps and Cents and Diabetes

A similar set of calculations can be used to examine potential relief strategies for diabetes costs.

Every prevented case of diabetes saves $11,000 in annual charges. There are 1.3 million new cases of diabetes per year and if 58% were prevented (as in the Diabetes Prevention Trial described previously) it would save $8.3 billion per year. If half of this number comes from increased activity it would lead to a figure of $4.2 billion of cost savings by preventing new cases. The amount of exercise in the studies is approximately 8 met hours per week, equivalent to two to three hours of walking.

If half of the prevention saving is attributable to the exercise part of the protocol, 30 steps saves 1 cent of diabetes cost.

These simple calculations based on the costs of diabetes and obesity emphasize the enormous amounts of money which can be saved not by expensive new technology, but by simply putting our bodies in motion and watching how many calories we eat.

Maybe we won't take care of ourselves simply because we should, but if it saves big bucks perhaps an additional motivation will kick in.

8

Changing Behavior Through IOI: Information, Opportunity, and Incentive

In the first chapter, I proposed that the present threat to mankind's future is one of the direst in our entire time as a species on this planet. I suggested that this crisis was totally unforeseen just a few years ago. Until yesterday, diabetes was only a small blip on the radar screen. What happened so fast?

Historical review reveals that our biology hasn't changed in all this time. We are faithful reproductions of our hunter-gatherer ancestors who deeded us their complete set of fit and lean genes. Our genes allowed our species to survive the many perils which they confronted and overcame.

We have survived and even thrived despite huge adversities—initially starvation and more recently infection. All this has changed. Now we are in an era of collective suicide, dying slow deaths at our own hands. Our suicide weapon of diabetes exploits our own genetic vulnerability to avoid movement, unless threatened, and to try to slake our historical hunger by supersizing, all at one sitting.

We eat too much, we move too little, and we live too fast.

We now can characterize our biology with great precision. We know every component of our body's carbon, hydrogen, nitrogen, oxygen, phosphorus, sulfur mixture. We know how these elements miraculously come together to cause our bodies to function with extraordinary fidelity. We know our micro-anatomy and micro-physiology at every level.

Yet we have forsaken our primitive advantage. We have abandoned the very shaping environmental forces that created us in the first place: hunger and movement.

Now we move too little. We eat too much, and we live too fast.

We are the most adaptive of the world's species. We live high and low. We live north, south, east, and west. We live young and old. We live hot and cold. We live dry and wet. Our glorious bodies can absorb a lot of abuse, but even they have a breaking point. When balance is distorted by progressive excesses and deficiencies, we struggle to maintain control.

The robustness of our species is tested by our own institutions, borne out of the capitalist society which we have created and embraced. It is our organizing vehicle for getting us through life, and despite its own excesses and deficiencies no one has yet figured out a better way. Capitalism works by providing its own set of checks and balances. If a product is good, make it or sell it or buy it. This calculation has seemed to turn out right most of the time.

But what if something we make is bad for us, even if it enriches us? And what if something we make is both bad for us and we like it?

Certain rules of capitalism have evolved. Thou shalt not cheat is a clear capitalist moral. Individual and corporate goals seem to have a way of sorting themselves out in capitalism. But what if what is good for General Motors is bad for America? Or what if what is good for GM and the soft-drink manufactures is bad for our biology? These companies and their stockholders, you and I, did not hold clandestine meetings to corrupt our biology, but historic forces have conspired to encourage us to move less, eat more, and live too fast.

The wheel and electricity, the two main tools of capitalism have uncoupled us from our primitive and well tested lifestyle.

But the human organism now faces an entirely new threat, for which our genes have not had the chance to declare their fitness.

In fact their fitness to encounter and overcome this environmental challenge is not only untested, but it appears to be part of the problem and therefore not part of the solution. When genes are ill-suited to the environment, disaster looms.

There is a lot of evidence that this mismatch is not just a local or temporary problem. It is universal and steadfast in its worsening. The roof is on fire. Smoke billows, yet we sleep. Wake up world!

Where can we turn for rescue? As stated repeatedly the fire department is not up to the job. The epidemic is too big. It is beyond a medical solution. I have no confidence in technical fixes when such primitive forces are in control.

How about dialing up the government and asking for their help in this mess? Like the corporate execs, our elected officials, our elite chosen leaders, whose depth of focus and attention span is measured in milliseconds and conformed strictly to their term in office, feel the heat only when they are being scorched. By this time, the opportunity for effective action has been lost. Governments around the world are burdened by expedient policies which are no longer defensible.

Our Failing Grades

Chapters 3 and 4 detailed the compelling insights provided by the Prevention and Control Studies. These impressive, conclusive studies provide a clear mandate for action-prevention and control. How are we doing? TERRIBLY!

We certainly aren't preventing. The diabetes inferno is spreading out of its bounds. And we certainly aren't controlling anything. All observations point to the fact that satisfactory control is an illusion across the globe. If we aren't preventing and we're not controlling, what are we doing? While smarter at the science level, while spending a lot of money, we are still failing. We deserve an F grade.

Where can we turn for rescue? In 2001, the Danish Pharmaceutical Company, Novo Nordisk, formed the international Diabetes Attitudes, Wishes, and Needs (DAWN) project. Leaders from 13 countries participated. They identified the F grade that our medical care model receives.

Five thousand four hundred and twenty-six adult diabetic patients were surveyed. Three thousand eight hundred professional care givers participated. They concluded that our medical model for diabetes is failing, despite its costs and intellectual capital, because of its focus on the disease instead of on the person who has the disease or is trying to catch it. Like Bandura, they recommend a vastly increased emphasis on the psychosocial components of diabetes. Until and unless the individual takes responsibility, we will continue to fail. The fire will burn brighter and more broadly.

Possible Strategies

Martin Luther King and Gandhi accomplished much by mobilizing civil discontent into political action. Could their strategies work for a diabetes solution? Could we hold up traffic on the Golden Gate Bridge, US 101, or disable golf carts and elevators to signal our non-acceptance of riding?

What about jailing those amongst us who even passively participate in Diabetes Doomsday? I have jokingly proposed serving arrest warrants to our local school principals who totally ignore California State mandates for 200 minutes of physical education every two weeks for our students. They can't get away with that. Can they?

What about boycott? Could we stop patronizing those products that participate in our burgeoning diabesity? This theoretically could work, but we find ourselves in the position of liking and buying the very products that are killing us. A boycott would have problems.

How about a class action suit brought on behalf of all the 200 million or so of us who move too little and eat too much, and live too fast? We certainly could qualify enough signatures. What about a general strike? What if we all collectively sat down and refused to move until something was done about our diabetes epidemic? Well, it is obvious that we're already doing just this, and it is making things worse. Strikes have a way of sometimes causing more problems than they settle.

Well if civil disobedience or prison or boycott or class action suits or a general strike are ruled out, what's left?

How about education? It is a perpetual amazement to me to recognize how unknowing we are to the diabetes danger. Despite great advances in scientific understanding of the disease, the public is largely ignorant. Procrastination or worse rules. I have been involved in hundreds of cases of diabetic mothers with fat kids who just don't have a clue as to what's going on.

Even doctors don't seem to grasp the intensity of this scourge consuming us. We seem to have adequate book learning, but writing a prescription is a feeble a way of addressing a disease with multiple, beyond-a-pill components.

Twenty years ago, a group at the Indiana University School of Medicine formed Diabetes Education Study (DIABEDS). It involved 532 Type 2 patients, mostly older African American women. It divided the group in half and monitored the improvement in knowledge and diabetes control in those who received the intensive instruction versus the controls.

A significant improvement in sugar levels, A1C levels, body weight, and blood pressure was found. As impressive as this study results were, the most important observation is how few other such efforts are published. There are hundreds of articles about drug treatment results, but only a few about the critical results of educational effort. Why?

Education is the absolute first line of attack to approach any problem. Logic is essential. How can you extinguish a blaze without knowing a fire exists?

Opportunities for Using Knowledge

But knowledge, while necessary, is insufficient. Moving too little, eating too much, living too fast are not always the only issues. If there is no decent, inexpensive food available, what happens? Or what if I want to take a walk and there's no safe place to take it? Do I instead stay home and watch TV? Or what if I'm working two jobs and have no time for my kids and wife, let alone my own health? Knowledge without the opportunity to endorse that knowledge is useless.

Knowledge plus Opportunity are Insufficient

But even with full knowledge and full opportunity, I propose that these two essentials are insufficient to douse the diabetes inferno without incentives. These incentives are money.

As things now stand, health and capitalism are ill-matched. Disease is very, very good for business. It is so good for business in America that it is draining our educational system of the means to pay for its teachers. Not only are we told that our generation of children is the first in the history of our republic that will live shorter lives than their parents, but on the same newscast we are told that for the first time in half a century our income as Americans is going down—not because we're making less money, but because we are being forced to spend more on our health care expenses than is matchable by increased productivity. Our national factory makes more widgets to increase profits, but diabetes costs siphon them from the assembly line faster than the workers can crank them out.

This collision of living less long and losing money in the bargain at the same time is unsustainable. This crash is right out there for all to see and feel as our individual and collective ways of life are being eroded.

As education and opportunity are insufficient by themselves we need incentives to help redesign our priorities.

I urge policymakers at every level to shuffle their priorities so that health can pay, and disease and the parlayers of disease become the bankroll, the financial engine for this revolutionary fork in the road. I urge the incenting of the payers of our $1.8 trillion annual disease bill to re-budget for health. There certainly is not a lack of funding. We are awash in health care spending. Lack of money is *not* the problem. Its distribution *is*.

We need to incentivize prevention so that we don't have to pay these huge costs after the fact.

Incentivize Prevention

For the diabetes danger to recede from its current rule of posing the threat of imminent extinction, we must collectively and individually come to grips with reality.

Making policy recommendations for improved diabetes care, the University of Michigan gave first priority to the payment inequity between a prevention strategy and the complications strategy, where most of the billions of diabetes cost are now being spent. We're not spending out dollars on the right things! Where is the endorsement of this vital concern?

John Gardner, former Secretary of Health, Education, and Welfare, often said, "We are faced directly with breathtaking opportunities disguised as insoluble problems."

Feeling Better, Costing Less

In March 2003, Arkansas's extremely popular governor, Mike Huckabee, weighed nearly 300 pounds and was told that he had diabetes. He had allowed slow diabetes to creep up on him, despite watching both of his parents suffer the torments of diabetes.

He recognized that he might not live long enough to finish his term as governor in 2007. After several futile unsupervised efforts, he sought help at the outstanding weight control program at the University of Arkansas for Medical Science. It worked. A year later, his XXXL clothing size had shrunk to L. His waist size reduced from 48 in. to 35 in. He had lost 105 pounds. To illustrate this, while visiting a local school in Little Rock, he hoisted a seventh grader over his shoulder like a sack of grain and paraded around the gym to show the cheering students the equivalent of how much weight he had lost.

As newsworthy as the governor's personal weight loss success is, it is dwarfed by the public-policy which he initiated as a result of his own life crisis.

As governor, he identified that his state was one of this country's unhealthiest. 235,000 other Arkansans also had diabetes. There was a 77% increase in obesity in ten years. Arkansas ranked first in stroke mortality.

The Medicaid program in Arkansas covers 600,000 people, 22% of the population. These persons cost the state $3 billion per year. The surge in Medicaid costs threatens both teachers' salaries and road repair. Seventy seven percent of the costs come from chronic diseases, the causes for which are poor fitness, poor diet, and cigarette smoking.

The governor looked into his mirror and didn't like what he saw. He recognized that his state was essentially in the same poor shape that he had been in, and it was costing them all big bucks. In May 2004, he launched "Healthy Arkansas—for a Better State of Health."

The program is inspired. It affects all levels, from the individual to the entire state. It is wide reaching and intended to incorporate every element in the state—from schools to industry to media, to government, to the medical system. For example, Huckabee introduced a program for all state employees to incentivize healthy behavior change. As the employee takes a voluntary health risk appraisal, he is rewarded by a $250 rebate on his health insurance premiums. Co-payments for preventive medical services are eliminated. These programs are slated to be extended to the teachers next year.

Huckabee encourages the employers in his state to embrace a wellness protocol by providing half-hour periods during the workday for physical activity. Employers already are realizing a 20% to 50% reduction in health care costs by pursuing these preventive strategies. Huckabee encourages media campaigns for competition between towns and companies, and awards are given for "The Healthiest." Programs encourage schools to undertake nutrition and physical activity encouragement. He establishes "hometown health leaders" to act as volunteer coordinators. The Veterans Health System Wellness Program saved $817,000 in its first year and demonstrated an 8 to 1 cost-benefit savings.

The Arkansas Diabetes Control Program was initiated in partnership with the Eli Lilly Company. Its efforts include a greatly expanded diabetes education program with diabetes educators focused in 24 low income education centers throughout the state.

Huckabee has certainly personally benefited. His diabetes seems to have gone away. Whether this is a honeymoon or a permanent cure, it is encouraged by his current vigorous physical regimen, arising early for a three-mile run followed by a stationary bike workout. He has reformulated his diet to eat a healthy diet, with lots of fruits, vegetables. He says "McDonalds' didn't cause my diabetes. I did."

Governor Huckabee is not alone among the nation's governors and leaders to target diabetes. Even President George W. Bush is an advocate. I personally wish that he were more vocal in his advisories, which he largely delegates to the Secretary of Health and Human Services, Surgeon General Carmona, and to the President's Council on Physical Activity and Sport. They use small megaphones. What we really need is the loudspeaker. We need our President to sound the alarm that Mike Huckabee is sounding. Until that happens, maybe we need to clone the Arkansas governor.

How Can We Reverse the Obesity Trend?

It is so important that parents get involved in assuring that food choices available at their children's school are nutritious. As I mentioned earlier, California, as well as some other states, have actually banned soda and unhealthy snacks from school vending machines.

Meals provided at schools should be evaluated for their nutritional benefit. While students must have some choices, is it reasonable to offer healthy foods rather than unhealthy high fat, high sugar foods? Can we assume our children are going to chose to eat the vegetables, baked chicken and whole wheat rolls if they are offered a hamburger, french fries, chocolate cake and soda?

We must also strongly advocate for our young people's physical education. We know physical activity is crucial in the prevention of obesity and many chronic diseases. School is an opportune time for children to develop a daily routine which includes physical activity. Providing a variety of physical activity options will also assist them in choosing an activity they can continue throughout their life. It also is an opportunity to learn the value of physical activity in maintaining health. Talking about physical activity and its value is not as effective as actually participating in physical activities and learning how they may be incorporated into your day.

Recently, a report showcased a company that provided a track in their meeting room; meetings took place as participants walked around the room. This company has treadmills in each office; employees can walk while using the computer. These are great, revolutionary steps. Maybe you've noticed that even airports are recognizing the value of providing facilities for travelers to exercise while waiting for flights.

Do these seem like drastic measures? Not to me. In order to reverse the obesity trend, we must make physical activity readily available.

Extinguishing the Diabetes Inferno

Diabetes may seem too big, too complex, too overwhelming to consider seeking a solution. However, the last several decades have witnessed two huge reversals of seeming disaster.

At one point, smoking seemed poised to eradicate us by causing lung cancer, despite the cigarette companies' shrieking denials of its dangers. But in just a few years, this evil scourge is in full retreat—due to a society-wide counterattack employing a host of creative strategies, some educational, some penal, and some fiscal. Billions of dollars and millions of lives are redistributed.

The second recent health revolution concerns heart disease. Despite its retaining the bragging rights of being number one killer, its relentless annual rate of increased incidence first slackened and is now reversed. It is 30-40% less prevalent now than when it was at its worst 15 years ago.

An important lesson to be learned comes from the Finnish region of North Karelia. In the 1960s and 1970s this community was identified as having the world's highest incidence of heart disease. Local leaders decided to act. By a combination of intensive community education, smoking prevention, diet modification, and the promotion of strong collective cohesion the heart disease mortality was reduced by 73%.

Program elements included workplace efforts to reduce weight, availability of vegetables in all stores, cooperative steps with local business leaders to promote healthy lifestyles, legislation to limit smoking, promotion of discussion groups on heart disease risk reduction, competition between communities to encourage physical activity, and other steps.

Again a multiplicity of factors contributes to this sigh of relief. The drop in smoking gets credit for one third of the improvement. Medical advances claim another third of the credit, while lifestyle improvements are responsible for the rest.

The major point of these two great reversals is how urgent was their cause, and how rapid has been the reaction. No one person or group sat down and crafted the grand strategy of counterattack. It arose out of the absolute necessity for solution. Necessity provoked the invention.

Diabetes now screams for solutions. For the answer to appear, multiple components will need to emerge. Certainly a massive distribution of knowledge is essential. Such knowledge needs to partner with opportunity for change. Knowledge and opportunity require the financial incentives, which our capitalistic society should be adept at crafting.

But knowledge, opportunity, and incentive are incomplete without will.

Until our unfit, overfed, speeded-up world recognizes the diabetes inferno now burning out of control, we are in tremendous peril. We must find the will to wake up, and put out the fire.

Recently I heard an address at the World Affairs' Council by Dr.Wangari Maathai, winner of the Nobel Peace Prize for 2004. This fine Kenyan woman is celebrated for her work with the Green Belt movement, which since 1977 has planted 30 million trees in Africa, where deforestation has wrought havoc and despair. She uses local approaches to frame environmental stewardship as a human rights issue.

During her address she told the following story of a fire. It seems that one fine day, smoke was seen rising from deep within the jungle. At first there was no alarm, but soon crackles were heard, flames leapt, and birds started to shriek. Slowly, the danger was perceived by all, and with wide eyes and tears they left their dens, perches, burrows and nests and started to run away. A path was clear to a large hill a short way outside of the jungle.

So the parrots and zebras and monkeys and snakes and elephants and toads all found their way to this lookout hill where they gathered to see their homes being consumed by pillars of fire. Much of their vision was obscured by billows of smoke. As they gazed numbly at the scene, the tortoise saw a tiny speck against the smoke, which at first he thought was a cinder. But he noted that it seemed to be purposeful in its course, repeatedly passing overhead.

The tortoise alerted the other animals to this dot. They collectively recognized this dot as a tiny hummingbird. This hummingbird was seen to emerge from the smoke and fly directly to their left to the river where it dipped down for a moment and returned immediately into the smoke and flames. All the animals wondered at this tiny sight.

One called out, "Sister Hummingbird, what are you doing? You know that you can't put out the fire with just a tiny amount of water."

To which the hummingbird replied. "I'm just doing the best I can."

To me this is the perfect parable for our diabetes danger. If, individually and collectively, we do the best we can, then not even this huge blaze can withstand our efforts.

Appendix A

All About Vision
Information is provided on eye health, vision correction options, and low vision adaptive devices.

http://www.allaboutvision.com

American Association of Clinical Endocrinologists
Guidelines for the management of diabetes are available as well as a listing of endocrinologists in the United States.

904-353-7878   http://www.aace.com

American Association of Diabetes Educators
A listing of diabetes educators is provided by zip code.

800-832-6874   http://www.diabeteseducator.org

American Association of Kidney Patients
Serve the needs, interests and welfare of all kidney patients and their families. Its mission is to improve the lives of fellow kidney patients and their families by helping them to deal with the physical, emotional and social impact of kidney disease.

800-636-8100   http://www.aakp.org

American Diabetes Association
Offers information on diabetes care for patients and health professionals, provides a listing of diabetes self-management programs and advocates for individuals with diabetes.

800-DIABETES   http://www.diabetes.org

American Dietetic Association
Provides information on how a dietitian can help you learn about healthy eating.

800-877-1600   http://www.eatright.org

American Heart Association
Information is provided on heart disease, cholesterol, and stroke.

800-242-8721   http://www.americanheart.org

Be Smart About Your Heart: Control the ABC's of Diabetes
Information is provided to increase awareness of the risk of heart disease and stroke. Also offers tips on controlling blood glucose, blood pressure and lowering cholesterol.

                        http://www.ndep.nih.gov/campaigns/
                        BeSmart/BeSmart_index.htm

Canadian Diabetes Association
Provides information on its divisions and branches in Canada and has articles about diabetes and new developments in treatment.
800-832-6874   http://www.diabetes.ca

Centers for Disease Control—Diabetes Home Page
Provides information to improve the health of people with diabetes and gathers statistical data regarding the prevalence of diabetes and its complications.

877-CDC-DIAB   http://www.cdc.gov/diabetes

CenterWatch Clinical Trials Listing Service
A listing of ongoing clinical research trials is provided. Use this listing to search for clinical trials, find out information about physicians and medical centers performing clinical research, and learn about drug therapies recently approved by the Food and Drug Administration.

800-765-9647   http://www.centerwatch.com

Children with Diabetes

This site promotes understanding of the care and treatment of diabetes, especially in children. A comprehensive index provides information on a variety of products, computerized programs for diabetes management, resources, and educational materials.

http://www.childrenwithdiabetes.com

Diabetes at Work

Developed in conjunction with the National Diabetes Education program this site assists businesses in the development of programs dealing with the diabetes epidemic.

http://www.diabetesatwork.org

Diabetes Mall

This site provides forums on diabetes topics, information on insulin pumps and self-management tools.

800-988-4772   http://www.diabetesnet.com

Diabetes Monitor

Offers educational forums, question and answers and current information about diabetes, this is a resource for patients to educate themselves about their role as active participants in their care.

http://www.diabetesmonitor.com

DiabetesPortal.com

Provides information about advanced treatments for insulin-dependent diabetes and to improve access to these treatments.

http://www.diabetesportal.com

Diabetes Research and Wellness Foundation

Provides free identification necklaces, ID cards and car decals "Please test my blood sugar" Provides educational materials and a toll-free helpline.

800-941-4635   http://www.drwf.org

Diabetes Research Institute
A world-recognized diabetes research institute located at the University of Miami.

800-321-3437   http://www.drinet.org

Diabetic Exercise and Sports Association
DESA exists to enhance the quality of life for people with diabetes through exercise and physical fitness.

800-898-4322   http://www.diabetes-exercise.org

Diabetes Institute for Immunology and Transplantation, University of Minnesota
A research facility which is seeking to develop and implement cures for diabetes through the disciplines of transplantation and immunology.

612-626-3016   http://www.diabetesinstitute.org

Drug Digest
This site provides informational materials on drugs, vitamins, herbs, drug interactions.

http://www.drugdigest.org

Feet for Life
Foot care is vital for diabetics. The Society of Chiropodists and Podiatrists web site offers tips and information to help prevent common foot problems.

http://www.feetforlife.org

50+ Lifelong Fitness
This website encourages a healthy life-style for individuals over 50.

http://www.50plus.org

Gastroparesis and Dysmotilities Association
This site raises awareness of gastroparesis through education and advocacy.

http://www.gpda.net

Insulin Free World Foundation
This site is devoted to helping people to find ways—not to manage, not to live with—but to overcome diabetes.
http:///www.insulin-free.org/

Insulin Pumpers Support Group
This site provides a support system for individuals using the insulin pump.
http://www.insulin-pumpers.org

International Association for Medical Assistance to Travelers
A non-profit organization advises travelers about health risks, immunization requirements for all countries, and lists resources for medical care available to travelers by western-trained doctors who speak English.
716-754-4883   http://www.iamat.org

International Diabetes Federation (IDF)
This non-governmental organization acts as a global advocate for people with diabetes to promote care, prevention and a cure for diabetes worldwide.
http://www.idf.org

Joslin Diabetes Center
Joslin is a premier diabetes care center, that provides information to improve the lives of people with diabetes and its complications through innovative care, education and research.
617-732-2400   http://www.joslin.org

Juvenile Diabetes Foundation
This organization raises funds for the development of innovative therapies which will result in a cure for diabetes.
800-533-2873   http://www.jdf.org

Medline Plus
A joint effort of the National Library of Medicine and the National Institute of Health to provide educational materials on over 700 health topics—articles, tutorials, pictures, and graphics.
http://www.medlineplus.gov

David Mendosa Diabetes Directory
A comprehensive list of resources on all aspects of diabetes self-management can be found on this site.

http://www.mendosa.com/diabetes

National Diabetes Education Program
A joint effort of the National Institute of Health and the Centers for Disease Control provides culturally sensitive information on controlling and preventing diabetes.

800-860-8747   http://www.ndep.nih.gov

National Eye Institute
Conducts and supports research that helps prevent and treat eye diseases and other disorders of vision.

301-496-5248   http://www.nei.nih.gov

National Federation for the Blind
An organization that provides resources for individuals with diabetes who are blind or have vision loss.

410-659-9314   http://www.nfb.org/diabetes.htm

National Institute of Diabetes and Digestive and Kidney Diseases
Conducts and supports research on diabetes and kidney diseases affecting public health.

http://www.niddk.nih.gov

National Kidney Disease Educational Program
This site provides educational information on kidney disease.

http://www.nkdep.nih.gov

Neuropathy Association
This organization offers information and resources for individuals suffering from neuropathy.

212-692-0662   http://www.neuropathy.org

New York Online Access to Health (NOAH)
This website provides a variety of educational information on diabetes and a variety of health conditions.

http://www.noah-health.org

NutritionData

This site offers nutrition facts, calorie counts, and nutrient data for all foods and recipes.

http://www.nutritiondata.com

Simple Steps to Dental Health

The Columbia University School of Dental and Oral Surgery offers dental health information.

http://www.simplestepsdental.com

Small Steps Big Rewards Prevent Type 2 Diabetes

Provides tools to lose weight and increase physical activity.

http://www.ndep.nih.gov/
campaigns/SmallSteps/
SmallSteps_index.htm

Steps to a Healthier US

A community initiative established to assist with the development of healthier lifestyles.

http://www.healthierus.gov

TOPS Club, Inc

A national organization offers a weight loss support group.

http://www.tops.org

United States Food and Drug Administration Diabetes Information

This site provides information on diabetes and diabetes medications.

http://www.fda.gov/diabetes

USDA 2005 Dietary Guidelines

Interactive website to assist you in following the 2005 dietary guidelines.

http://www.mypyramid.gov

Weight-control Information Network

This site provided by the National Institutes of Health offers up-to-date, science-based health information on weight control, obesity, physical activity, and related nutritional issues.

877-946-4627   http://www.win.niddk.
                            nih.gov/index.htm

Weight Watchers

A weight loss support group available on-line or at locations throughout the United States.

800-978-2400   http://www.weightwatchers.com

Appendix B

Figure 24. **BODY MASS INDEX TABLE**

	Normal						Overweight					Obese						
BMI	19	20	21	22	23	24	25	26	27	28	29	30	31	32	33	34	35	36
Height (inches)							Body Weight (pounds)											
58	91	96	100	105	110	115	119	124	129	134	138	143	148	153	158	162	172	177
59	94	99	104	109	114	119	124	128	133	138	143	148	153	158	163	168	173	178
60	97	102	107	112	118	123	128	133	138	143	148	153	158	163	168	174	179	184
61	100	106	111	116	122	127	132	137	143	148	153	158	164	169	174	180	185	190
62	104	108	115	120	126	131	136	142	147	153	158	164	169	175	180	186	191	196
63	107	113	118	124	130	135	141	146	152	158	163	169	175	180	186	191	197	203
64	110	116	122	128	134	140	145	151	157	163	169	174	180	186	192	197	204	209
65	114	120	126	132	138	144	150	156	162	168	174	180	186	192	198	204	210	216
66	118	124	130	136	142	148	155	161	167	173	179	186	192	198	204	210	216	223
67	121	127	134	140	146	153	159	166	172	178	185	191	198	204	211	217	223	230
68	125	131	138	144	151	158	164	171	177	184	190	197	203	210	216	223	230	236
69	128	135	142	149	155	162	169	176	182	189	196	203	209	216	223	230	236	243
70	132	139	146	163	160	167	174	181	188	195	202	209	216	222	229	236	243	250
71	136	143	150	157	165	172	179	186	193	200	208	215	222	229	236	243	250	257
72	140	147	154	162	169	177	184	191	199	206	213	221	228	235	242	250	258	265
73	144	151	159	166	174	182	189	197	204	212	219	227	235	242	250	257	265	272
74	148	155	163	171	179	186	194	202	210	218	225	233	241	249	256	264	272	280
75	152	160	168	176	184	192	200	208	216	224	232	240	248	256	264	272	279	287
76	156	164	172	180	189	197	205	213	221	230	238	246	254	263	271	279	287	295

BODY MASS INDEX TABLE (Cont.)

	Obese			Extreme Obesity															
BMI	37	38	39	40	41	42	43	44	45	46	47	48	49	50	51	52	53	54
Height (inches)							Body Weight (pounds)											
58	177	181	186	191	196	201	205	240	215	220	224	229	234	239	244	248	253	258
59	183	188	193	198	203	208	212	217	222	227	232	237	242	247	252	257	262	267
60	189	194	199	204	209	215	220	225	230	235	240	245	250	255	261	266	271	276
61	195	201	206	211	217	222	227	232	238	243	248	254	259	264	269	275	280	285
62	202	207	213	218	224	229	235	240	246	251	256	262	267	273	278	284	289	295
63	208	214	220	225	231	237	242	248	254	259	265	270	278	282	287	293	299	304
64	215	221	227	232	238	244	250	256	262	267	273	279	285	2714296	302	308	314
65	222	228	234	240	246	252	258	264	270	276	282	288	294	300	306	312	318	324
66	229	235	241	247	253	260	266	272	278	284	291	297	303	309	305	322	328	334
67	236	242	249	255	261	268	274	280	287	293	299	306	312	319	325	331	338	344
68	243	249	256	262	269	276	282	289	295	302	308	315	322	328	335	341	348	354
69	250	257	263	270	277	284	291	297	304	311	318	324	331	338	345	351	358	365
70	257	264	271	278	285	292	298	306	313	320	327	334	341	348	355	362	369	376
71	265	272	279	286	293	301	308	315	322	329	338	343	351	358	365	372	379	386
72	272	279	287	294	302	309	316	324	331	338	346	353	361	368	375	383	390	397
73	280	288	295	302	310	318	325	333	340	348	355	363	371	378	386	393	401	408
74	287	295	303	311	319	326	334	342	350	358	365	373	381	389	396	404	412	420
75	295	303	311	319	327	335	343	351	359	367	375	383	391	399	407	415	423	431
76	304	312	320	328	336	344	353	361	369	377	385	394	402	410	418	426	435	443

Index